OTHER BOOKS BY DR. MERCOLA

Gut Cure: Stop the Rot: Restore Your Body from the Inside Out (2026)

Your Guide to Cellular Health: Unlocking the Science of Longevity and Joy (2024)

The Truth About COVID-19: Exposing the Great Reset, Lockdowns, Vaccine Passports, and the New Normal (2021, with Ronnie Cummins)

*EMF*D: 5G, Wi-Fi & Cell Phones: Hidden Harms and How to Protect Yourself* (2020)

KetoFast: Rejuvenate Your Health with a Step-by-Step Guide to Timing Your Ketogenic Meals (2019)

Fat for Fuel: A Revolutionary Diet to Combat Cancer, Boost Brain Power, and Increase Your Energy (2017)

Effortless Healing: 9 Simple Ways to Sidestep Illness, Shed Excess Weight, and Help Your Body Fix Itself (2015)

Dark Deception: Discover the Truths About the Benefits of Sunlight Exposure (2008)

Generation XL: Raising Healthy, Intelligent Kids in a High-Tech, Junk-Food World (2007)

Take Control of Your Health (2007, with Dr. Kendra Degen Pearsall)

The Great Bird Flu Hoax: The Truth They Don't Want You to Know About the "Next Big Pandemic" (2006, with Pam Killeen)

Sweet Deception: Why Splenda, NutraSweet, and the FDA May Be Hazardous to Your Health (2006, with Dr. Kendra Degen Pearsall)

The No-Grain Diet: Conquer Carbohydrate Addiction and Stay Slim for Life (2003, with Dr. Alison Rose Levy)

WEIGHT LOSS CURE

MELT FAT NATURALLY

With Your Own GLP-1

WEIGHT LOSS CURE

MELT FAT NATURALLY

With Your Own GLP-1

Dr. Mercola

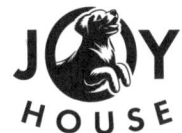

No portion of this book may be reproduced in any fashion, print, facsimile, or electronic, or by any method yet to be developed, without the express written permission of the publisher.

All images are proprietary. No use without written consent of Joy House Publishing. All rights reserved.

Take Control of Your Health is a registered trademark of Domain Technologies, LLC.

Hardcover ISBN: 978-1-965429-10-5

ebook ISBN: 978-1-965429-11-2

PUBLISHED BY
Joy House Publishing
125 SW 3rd Place, Suite 200
Cape Coral, FL 33991

Joyhousepublishing.com
For rights and permissions please contact media@mercola.com

Book and cover design by Alexia Garaventa

Manufactured in the United States of America

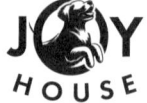

CONTENTS

Note to Readers ix

Quick-Start Guide xi

Introduction xxiii

CHAPTER 1 | 1
Weight-Loss Breakthroughs:
From Miracle Meds to Microbiome Magic

CHAPTER 2 | 35
GLP-1 Drugs: A Consumer-Friendly Blueprint

CHAPTER 3 | 59
The Origin Story of Akker

CHAPTER 4 | 79
Colonocytes, Gut Gems, and Your Gut Barrier

CHAPTER 5 | 95
The Seed-Oil Catastrophe:
How Seed Oils Changed Your Gut's Ecosystem

CHAPTER 6 | 113
GLP-1 and Akker's Secret Weapon

CHAPTER 7 | 131
How Dead Probiotics Help You Lose Weight

CHAPTER 8 | 150
The Fiber Paradox

CHAPTER 9 | 167
A Two-Step Restoration Protocol

CONCLUSION | 185

References 189

List of Figures 245

Index 249

Note to Readers

The author of this book does not advocate the use of any particular form of health care for all individuals but believes that the facts, figures, and knowledge presented herein should be available to every person concerned with improving his or her state of health. This book is not intended to replace the advice and treatment of the reader's personal physician or health-care provider. Any use of the information set forth herein is entirely at the reader's discretion.

The author and publisher are not responsible for any adverse effects or consequences resulting from the use of any of the preparations or procedures described in this book. This book is based upon the author's own opinion and theories. The reader should always consult with his or her own health-care practitioner before taking any medicine or dietary, nutritional, herbal, or homeopathic supplement, or beginning or stopping any therapy. The author is not intending to provide a substitute for the reader's personal medical advice and makes no warranty whatsoever, expressed or implied, with respect to any product, device, or therapy. No statement in this book has been reviewed or approved by the United States Food and Drug Administration or the Federal Trade Commission. Readers should use their own judgment in consultation with a holistic medical expert or their personal physician or health-care provider for specific applications to their health-care needs.

QUICK-START GUIDE
Weight Loss Cure: Reboot Your Gut, Reclaim Your Health

What you're about to read in these first few pages is a streamlined Quick-Start Guide—a condensed version of the book that gives you "the skinny up front." The key take-home points from each chapter are highlighted here so you can grasp the big picture quickly. The complete book goes much deeper, with detailed explanations, science, stories, and step-by-step guidance. If you want to take an even deeper dive, you'll also find a dedicated "professional" section at the end. That's where all of the references and source material live, so you can explore the research behind every recommendation. Think of this guide as your preview or road map: You'll get the essentials now, and you can always explore the full chapters and references for the nitty-gritty details.

INTRODUCTION
Miracle or Mirage?
These days, everyone seems to be talking about a new "miracle" for weight loss: weekly shots like Ozempic and Wegovy. You see them on TV and hear about them in the news. It sounds like a dream come true, a quick fix to melt away fat. But a closer look reveals that these meds may not be the miracle they're touted

as. For one thing, these shots can cause rough side effects, such as nausea and fatigue. They're expensive, and as soon as you stop taking them, the weight often comes right back. This book shows you a better way. We're going to focus on something most people ignore: your gut.

What happens in your intestines might be the missing piece of the weight-loss puzzle. Our modern diets—packed with ultra-processed foods and cheap vegetable oils (seed oils)—have damaged many people's gut health. If you've been eating the standard American diet (SAD), your gut might be paying the price.

Processed foods and vegetable oils weaken the protective lining of the gut and throw your bacterial community out of balance. The result is a slow-burning fire of inflammation inside you. When your body is inflamed, and your gut isn't healthy, it's easier to gain weight and harder to lose it. By repairing your gut and bringing your inner ecosystem back into balance, you can tackle the problem at its source.

Obesity and its health complications are more common than ever. But you have more control than you might think. This book is your guide to reclaiming that control by healing your gut and boosting the good bacteria that live there. It's about turning the "miracle cure" you've been searching for into something real and lasting—not a Band-Aid, but a true fix from within. So, let's get started on this journey from the questionable promise of miracle meds to the real deal: a healthy microbiome.

CHAPTER 1

Weight-Loss Breakthroughs: From Miracle Meds to Microbiome Magic

Drugs like Ozempic or Wegovy have become the new face of weight loss. They quiet hunger, deliver quick results, and sound almost magical. But there's a catch. Most people plateau after losing 10 to 15 percent of their body weight, and the pounds often return once the shots stop. Add in side effects and steep monthly costs, and the "miracle" starts to fade.

Here's the good news: Your gut already holds a powerful partner in weight control. *Akkermansia muciniphila*—nicknamed Akker in this book—strengthens the gut lining, supports other beneficial microbes, and helps regulate appetite and blood sugar. People with more Akker often stay leaner and metabolically healthier. Even pasteurized (heat-killed) Akker can deliver benefits, showing that its effects don't depend on live bacteria.

Quick fixes rarely last, but gut health can. By restoring balance in your microbiome, you set the stage for lasting energy, weight control, and resilience long after the hype of injections wears off.

CHAPTER 2

GLP-1 Drugs: A Consumer-Friendly Blueprint

Ozempic, Wegovy, and Mounjaro are hailed by stars and influencers as miracle fixes. These "skinny shots" seem to switch hunger off overnight. On GLP-1s, digestion slows so food stays in your stomach longer, helping you feel full. They also act on brain circuits to quiet cravings. But there are trade-offs. Common side effects include nausea, diarrhea, constipation, and that gaunt look nicknamed "Ozempic face." Less common but more serious are gallstones, stomach paralysis, and pancreatitis. Some even notice mood shifts, describing life as a bit "muted."

The other gut punch is cost. At $1,000 or more a month without coverage, it can quickly outweigh the benefit. Counterfeit versions have popped up, too—some risky, some ineffective.

If you and your doctor opt for these meds, think of them as scaffolding—temporary support while you build better habits. That way, you protect muscle and metabolism. Or skip the shots altogether and stick with proven basics: whole foods, daily activity, and consistency.

CHAPTER 3
The Origin Story of Akker

Back in the early 1900s, Élie Metchnikoff observed that Bulgarian villagers who ate lots of yogurt and kefir often lived longer. He believed lactic acid bacteria could crowd out harmful microbes and improve health. His ideas laid the foundation for probiotics, even though many beneficial bacteria, including Akker, weren't discovered until much later.

Before the early 2000s, scientists primarily studied microbes that could grow in air on lab plates. Anaerobic bacteria such as Akker stayed hidden because they couldn't survive those conditions. That meant much of the gut's real ecosystem remained invisible, and our picture of gut health was incomplete.

Akker makes its home in your gut's mucus layer, the very barrier designed to protect you. By feeding on mucus, it strengthens the gut lining, supports other beneficial microbes, and helps regulate your immune system. Research shows Akker boosts proteins that seal the gut barrier and promotes a calmer immune response, resulting in less inflammation and better metabolic health.

Around 2008, researchers began connecting the dots: People with more Akker were often leaner and had better blood sugar control. Akker quickly went from an obscure microbe to a key biomarker of a healthy gut. Today it's considered a front-runner in microbiome therapies and is even being studied as a potential tool against obesity, diabetes, and other metabolic conditions.

CHAPTER 4
Colonocytes, Gut Gems, and Your Gut Barrier

Colon cells (colonocytes) run best on a special fuel called butyrate. When they burn butyrate, they use up oxygen near the gut surface, creating the low-oxygen environment that microbes such as Akker need to thrive. A steady supply of butyrate means calmer digestion, stronger defenses, and a sturdier gut lining.

Butyrate and its partners—acetate and propionate—are short-chain fatty acids (SCFAs) that I've nicknamed "Gut Gems." Together they do more than energize cells: They act as signals that tighten the barrier, lower inflammation, and steady appetite hormones such as GLP-1 and PYY. When these signals are balanced, the gut lining stays sealed and the immune system works as it's supposed to.

Think of the gut barrier as a shield: It allows nutrients in while keeping irritants and toxins out. When the barrier weakens, fragments from food or bacteria can leak into your bloodstream, sounding alarms that drive up inflammation and strain metabolism. That's when risks such as insulin resistance, fatty liver, and weight gain increase.

You can reinforce your gut barrier with a few simple daily habits:

- **Ditch the seed oils.** Swap out soy, corn, sunflower, and safflower oils for butter, ghee, tallow, or coconut oil.

- **Tighten your eating window.** Aim to eat all your meals and snacks within an eight-to-ten-hour block each day to give your gut time to repair itself.

- **Walk it in.** Add thirty to sixty minutes of walking daily to stabilize blood sugar and support barrier strength.

CHAPTER 5

The Seed-Oil Catastrophe

Industrial seed oils—soy, corn, canola, sunflower, and others—permeate today's food supply. Marketed as "heart-healthy," they're cheap and built into almost every packaged or fried food. The problem? They're loaded with linoleic acid (LA), a fragile fat that easily breaks down under heat, light, and oxygen, creating toxic by-products that stress your gut.

When fragile fats are built into your gut lining, they weaken the barrier. Cell membranes grow unstable, inflammation builds, and the gut environment tips in favor of harmful microbes. Beneficial bacteria such as Akker struggle to survive, leaving irritation, imbalance, and leaks in the wall.

For decades, seed oils were promoted as healthier than butter or lard because they lower LDL cholesterol. But that guidance overlooked the gut. Today, LA overload is recognized as a hidden driver of chronic inflammation and metabolic disease. The fix starts with swaps: Check labels and cut back on foods where seed oils rank high on the ingredient list. For cooking, stick with stable options: olive oil for salads and low heat, tallow or coconut oil for high heat, and butter for baking and flavor. Traditional fats in moderation, paired with whole foods, help restore a resilient gut environment.

CHAPTER 6

GLP-1 and Akker's Secret Weapon

Deep in the intestine live L cells. This tiny but mighty group of cells make up less than 1 percent of the gut lining yet act as powerful nutrient sensors. When food passes by, they detect sugars, fats, and even the stretch of the gut wall.

Once triggered, L cells release hormones such as GLP-1 and PYY. Together, these messengers slow digestion, steady blood sugar, and tell your brain you're full. GLP-1 boosts insulin and delays stomach emptying, while PYY reinforces the slowdown, giving a comfortably satisfied feeling after a meal.

Here's where the gut ally Akker adds a secret edge. Akker produces proteins that act as natural, gentle mimics of weight-loss drugs. One example, P9, nudges L cells to release GLP-1 without flooding the whole system, unlike an injection, and with far fewer side effects. Even pasteurized (heat-killed) Akker works because its proteins keep sending positive signals.

Quick Start Guide

The good news is you don't need shots to tap into this system. You can nurture it naturally:

- **Boost Akker.** Encourage growth with prebiotic-rich foods—chicory root, Jerusalem artichokes, onions, green bananas, and cooked-then-cooled potatoes or rice. Supplements with live or pasteurized Akker are also emerging.

- **Feed the gut.** Support mucus production and fiber fermentation with daily prebiotics.

- **Go protein forward.** Lean proteins such as fish, chicken, and Greek yogurt boost GLP-1 and PYY release while protecting muscle.

- **Add resistance training.** Building muscle improves blood sugar control and releases IL-6, a hormone that prompts L cells to boost GLP-1 naturally.

CHAPTER 7
How Dead Probiotics Help You Lose Weight

Similar to how vaccines train your immune system with pieces of a germ, postbiotics use parts of heat-killed (pasteurized) friendly bacteria to steer your body toward health. Your system recognizes their molecular "fingerprints" and responds as if to allies, strengthening the gut barrier, calming inflammation, and improving metabolism. So, probiotics don't have to be alive to work; they just have to deliver the right signals to your gut lining and immune system.

Postbiotics have unique advantages:

- **They're safe.** There's no risk of overgrowth; and they're good for sensitive or immunocompromised people.

- **They're stable.** No refrigeration is needed; and they tolerate travel and storage.

- **They're acid-proof.** They survive stomach acid and can act directly on the gut lining.
- **They're predictable.** They're a defined signal, not a finicky organism that may or may not take hold.

Akker is a rising star for gut and metabolic health. Even when pasteurized, it retains benefits. Its surface proteins and extracellular vesicles keep signaling your gut to strengthen the mucus layer, tighten junctions, and cool inflammation. In small human trials, pasteurized Akker improved insulin sensitivity, lowered fasting insulin, reduced cholesterol, and produced modest weight loss. It even outperformed live Akker.

Together these insights translate into a simple two-phase game plan. First, you lay the groundwork by calming inflammation and shoring up your gut barrier. Once that foundation is set, you layer in the foods and habits that help your microbes—and your metabolism—thrive:

- **Phase 1: Repair gut with postbiotic signals.** Add a pasteurized Akker supplement while removing seed oils and focusing on daily walking. This calms inflammation and rebuilds your barrier.
- **Phase 2: Rebuild with food.** Once the barrier is strengthened, layer in prebiotic-rich foods—chicory root, Jerusalem artichokes, onions, green bananas, and cooked-then-cooled rice or potatoes—to feed your microbes. Support with protein-forward meals and resistance training to amplify natural GLP-1 release.

Once you've laid the foundation with postbiotic signals and barrier repair, the next step is carefully choosing the right fuel. That's where chapter 8 picks up. Fiber is often hailed as the ultimate gut food, but timing and type matter. Without a strong barrier, even "healthy" fiber can backfire.

CHAPTER 8
The Fiber Paradox

Your gut is home to a bustling city of microbes, each with its own food preference. Some thrive on the gel-like fiber in oats, others on the crunch of veggie skins. When you serve up a variety of fibers, you feed more good bugs and create functional redundancy—if one species falters, another steps in. This diversity strengthens the gut barrier, lowers oxidative stress, and creates the oxygen-free zone microbes like Akker need to thrive.

If your gut lining is weak or inflamed, even "healthy" fiber can backfire. Instead of feeding only the friendly microbes, fermentable fiber can fuel opportunists. They ferment too quickly, causing gas, bloating, and irritation. Worse, bacterial fragments such as lipopolysaccharide (LPS, an endotoxin) can slip through the barrier and set off immune alarms. The cycle: more leakiness, more inflammation, and more metabolic strain. That's why barrier repair comes first.

Additionally, not all fiber works the same way. Each type plays a different role:

- **Soluble fiber** (oats, beans, fruit) forms a gel, slows glucose absorption, binds cholesterol, and ferments into Gut Gems such as butyrate.
- **Insoluble fiber** (whole grains, veggie skins) adds bulk, speeds transit, and helps prevent constipation.
- **Resistant starch** (green bananas, cooked-then-cooled potatoes or rice, lentils) escapes digestion and feeds butyrate-producing microbes.
- **Hemicelluloses** (rice bran, whole grains) need microbial teamwork to break down, which boosts mucus and diversity.

Together these types form a safety net for digestion, barrier health, and metabolism.

That said, fiber works best with a partner: polyphenols, the colorful compounds in berries, tea, coffee, cocoa, and spices. Polyphenols feed helpful microbes, suppress troublemakers, and reduce oxidative stress. They also encourage Akker to bloom, which thickens the mucus layer and reinforces the barrier. Pairing fiber with polyphenols strengthens your gut environment, naturally supporting GLP-1 and PYY signaling. Instead of relying on injections to dull hunger, you're amplifying your body's built-in appetite regulation.

To make fiber work for you:

- **Start slow.** Add about 5 grams per week to avoid bloating.
- **Choose gentler fibers first.** Cooked carrots, zucchini, ripe bananas, and oats are easier starters than raw kale or bran.
- **Stay hydrated.** Fiber acts like a sponge; water keeps things moving.
- **Pair with protein and color.** Protein helps your gut lining regenerate, while colorful polyphenols from berries, tea, or spices reinforce fiber's benefits and boost Akker.

With steady habits and gradual increases, you'll build a diverse, resilient microbiome that strengthens your gut barrier, steadies appetite, and fuels lasting metabolic health.

CHAPTER 9
A Two-Step Restoration Protocol

Think of your gut like a garden: You can't just scatter seeds and expect them to grow. First, you prepare the soil. In the gut that means repairing the barrier and cooling inflammation so new microbes can thrive. Only then do you add the "helpers"—live bacteria and the foods that keep them strong.

Phase 1: Barrier Repair (Weeks 0–4)
Start by removing irritants and strengthening the gut lining:

- **Cut fragile fats.** Minimize seed oils such as soybean, corn, and canola. Their unstable linoleic acid damages cell membranes and mucus.
- **Use a postbiotic.** Pasteurized Akker helps repair tight junctions in your gut lining, thicken mucus, and lower inflammation.
- **Lock in basics.** Sleep seven to eight hours each night, walk daily (thirty to sixty minutes, especially after meals), manage stress, and stay hydrated.

What to expect by week 4: less bloating, steadier energy, and more regular digestion. If progress is slow, extend this phase by another week or two before moving on.

Phase 2: Reseed and Rebuild (Weeks 4–12)
Once the barrier is calmer, add reinforcements:

- **Introduce live Akker.** Look for a product designed to survive the digestive tract.
- **Boost fiber diversity.** Gradually increase soluble, insoluble, resistant starch, and hemicelluloses. Start with gentle options such as oats or cooked veggies.
- **Add polyphenols daily.** Berries, tea, cocoa, herbs, and spices lower oxidative stress and support Akker.
- **Stay protein-forward.** Prioritize protein at breakfast and lunch to stabilize appetite and protect lean mass.

By week 12: Expect a thicker mucus layer, tighter junctions, calmer inflammation, and stronger satiety signals.

Keep tabs on your progress by tracking:

- Waist size, energy, and digestion (aim for Bristol Stool Form Scale types 3–4)
- Glucose markers if available (you want fasting glucose in the range of 80-89 mg/dL)

- Signs of reduced inflammation (fewer sugar crashes, steadier mood)

If stress, travel, or illness throw you off, run a short phase 1 "reset" for one week, then resume phase 2 habits.

Bottom line: Repair first, then reseed. Cut fragile fats, add a postbiotic signal, and build a diverse, fiber-plus-polyphenol plate. You'll reinforce the barrier, steady your appetite from the inside out, and create a metabolic rhythm you can sustain.

INTRODUCTION
The Weight-Loss Industry Needs a Gut Revolution

Weight loss today has a new face: the weekly shot. Ozempic, Wegovy, Mounjaro—these drugs have leapt from endocrinology journals to TikTok feeds and family dinner tables. They promise what once seemed impossible: dramatic, sustained weight loss without surgery or constant hunger. People shed twenty, thirty, even fifty pounds in a matter of months. Celebrities call them "life-changing." Doctors hail them as breakthroughs.

But there is a catch. The price tag often exceeds $1,000 a month; and side effects range from nausea and muscle loss to more serious complications, including, in some cases, blindness. Even when weight-loss results are good, they tend to plateau after six months. And almost universally, when people stop the injections, the weight creeps back on.

The paradox is that these drugs mimic GLP-1, which is a natural hormone the body already makes. GLP-1 is your appetite's volume knob. When food enters the intestines, it signals your brain to slow down eating, helps your pancreas release insulin, and steadies your blood sugar. In other words, the "miracle" of GLP-1 injections is merely a synthetic version of something your gut is already wired to provide. This raises a question that reframes the entire weight-loss industry: If your body has this system built in, why not strengthen it instead of outsourcing it to a lifelong costly prescription?

For most of medical history, the gut was treated as little more than a digestive tube—food goes in, waste comes out. But the last two decades have rewritten the story, and the gut is now recognized as a metabolic organ as essential as the pancreas or thyroid.

Much of that power comes from the gut's inhabitants—trillions of microbes live along your intestinal lining, collectively called "the microbiome." These microbes are not freeloaders; they're chemical factories. They produce vitamins, modulate the immune system, and send metabolic signals that shape whether someone stores calories as fat or burns them for energy. One shy microbe in particular, discovered in 2004 in a Dutch lab, has become a rising star: *Akkermansia muciniphila* (nicknamed Akker in this book). Akker thrives in the mucus lining of your intestines. There, it trims old mucus, stimulates new mucus growth, and keeps the barrier between your gut and bloodstream strong. Those with more Akker tend to be leaner, more insulin-sensitive, and less inflamed. And in animal experiments, adding Akker reduced weight gain and improved blood sugar control, even when the mice ate a high-fat diet.

What makes Akker so powerful is not magic but chemistry. As it consumes mucus, it produces valuable short-chain fatty acids—what I've nicknamed "Gut Gems." These include butyrate, acetate, and propionate. Gut Gems fuel the cells lining your colon, tighten the barrier that prevents toxins from leaking into your bloodstream, and calm inflammation. Even more striking, Gut Gems prompt specialized L cells in your intestines to release GLP-1 and PYY, the same appetite-quieting hormones that these popular weight-loss injections are built on. The gut is actually hardwired to keep us lean, but changes in the modern diet have interfered with the gut's processes, and obesity and diabetes have become widespread.

Your body, in other words, already has the machinery to regulate hunger and blood sugar through the same mechanisms—naturally. The challenge is that modern living has broken the body's machinery that would catalyze GLP-1 and PPY production on its own.

The first problematic change is the rise of fragile fats in our modern diet. Industrial seed oils—soybean, corn, safflower, sunflower—flood today's processed foods. Marketed for decades as "heart-healthy vegetable oils," they are high in linoleic acid, a polyunsaturated fat that oxidizes easily. When heated or stored, it breaks down into toxic by-products that injure the colon's cells, weaken the mucus barrier, and spark inflammation. They even interfere with the cells' ability to burn butyrate, leaving more oxygen in the colon—a disaster for the oxygen-intolerant microbes we rely on for optimal health.

The second problem in our modern diet is a lack of fiber. Our ancestors ate dozens of plant fibers daily—roots, tubers, fruits, grains, legumes. Each type of fiber fed a different guild of microbes. Today, most people barely reach 15 grams a day, less than half of what is recommended. Without fiber, beneficial microbes starve, oxygen creeps into areas where it doesn't belong, and harmful bacteria thrive. Together, fragile fats and a lack of fiber create a vicious cycle: weaker barriers, leakier guts, higher inflammation, and relentless hunger, eroding the environment that nourishes Akker and its allies.

But there's a twist. Microbes don't have to be alive to help you. Postbiotics—the components of inactivated bacteria—still deliver benefits. In a landmark human trial, researchers gave overweight adults either live Akker, pasteurized (heat-killed) Akker, or a placebo. Surprisingly, the pasteurized group had the best results. Their insulin sensitivity improved by nearly 30 percent, they had lowered their cholesterol, and they lost a few pounds—even more than the group with live Akker.

That is because the heat-killed cells still carried surface proteins and tiny vesicles that acted as molecular messengers, instructing gut cells to release GLP-1, tighten junctions, and reduce inflammation. One protein in particular, Amuc_1100, can signal directly to receptors on gut cells to reinforce the barrier. P9, another protein, attaches to immune and intestinal cells to trigger GLP-1 release.

These bacterial proteins function much like natural versions of GLP-1 drugs but are gentler, more targeted, and free of most side effects. This insight reframes the entire probiotics industry. You don't necessarily need to colonize your gut with live microbes. You can deliver their beneficial signals and still reap the benefits.

Restoring your body's natural weight-loss mechanisms will mean cutting fragile fats that corrode the gut barrier and supporting the microbiome with fibers that keep them thriving. It will mean leveraging postbiotics—safe, stable microbial fragments that act like nature's medicine. And it will take simple lifestyle changes such as walking after meals, getting restorative sleep, and reducing stress, all of which help the gut reset. Drugs work only as long as you inject them; a resilient microbiome sustains you for life.

CHAPTER 1
Weight-Loss Breakthroughs: From Miracle Meds to Microbiome Magic

Weight loss has a new poster child: weekly shots—self-injections that promise to melt away pounds like magic. If you've heard of Ozempic or Wegovy, you know the hype—and more drugs like them are on the way. A neighbor of mine lost twenty-five pounds on Wegovy in just four months, and she wasn't hungry all the time. It sounded like a dream come true. But by month six, her progress had stalled, and she complained of constant nausea and a loss of energy—no "spark." It's a common trade-off. Still worth it? You want the shortcut, but you don't want the toll booth. Before you start celebrating, you should be aware of the fine print.

These drugs are GLP-1 agonists, meaning they mimic a natural hormone in your body called glucagon-like peptide-1 (GLP-1).[1] Think of GLP-1 as your appetite's volume knob—useful when dinner sounds like a rock concert. Here's how it works: GLP-1 signals your brain that you're full,[2] slows down your stomach from emptying so you feel satisfied longer, and helps your pancreas release insulin to control blood sugar.[3] It's like turning down the dial on hunger and switching on your body's post-meal chill mode. No wonder people eat less and lose weight on these shots!

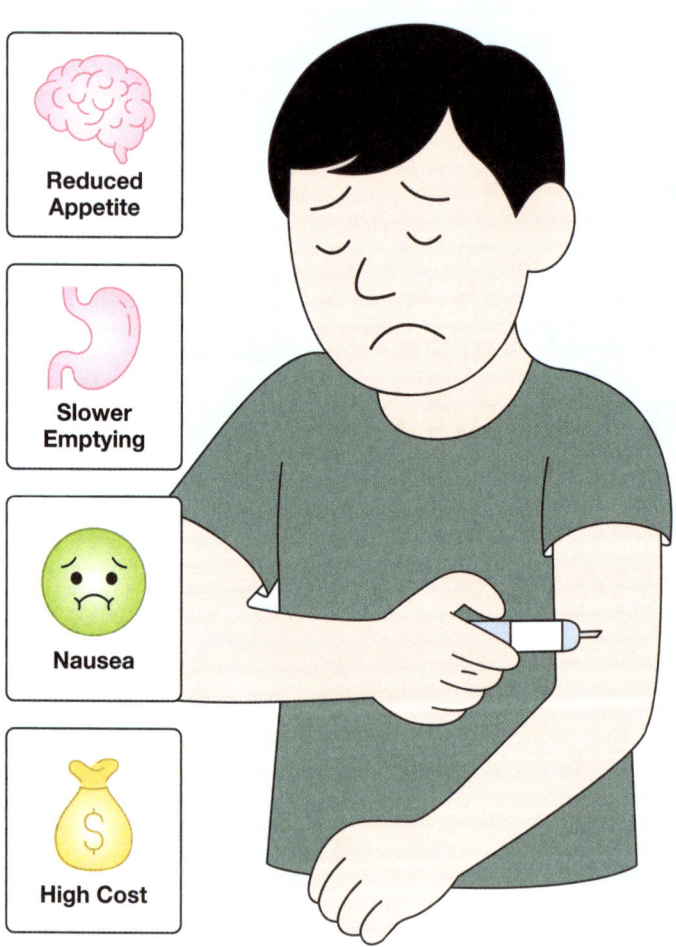

Figure 1. GLP-1 drugs hush hunger and slow the exit ramp from your stomach —handy, but the ticket price can include nausea and a heart-stopping pharmacy bill.

Sure, the first few months can feel miraculous, but then comes the plateau—for many, weight loss tapers off and eventually stagnates at around 10–15 percent of weight lost. If you stop the injections? Expect to regain most of the weight you lost within a year. In plain language, unless you make other changes or stay on the medication indefinitely, the pounds often creep back.

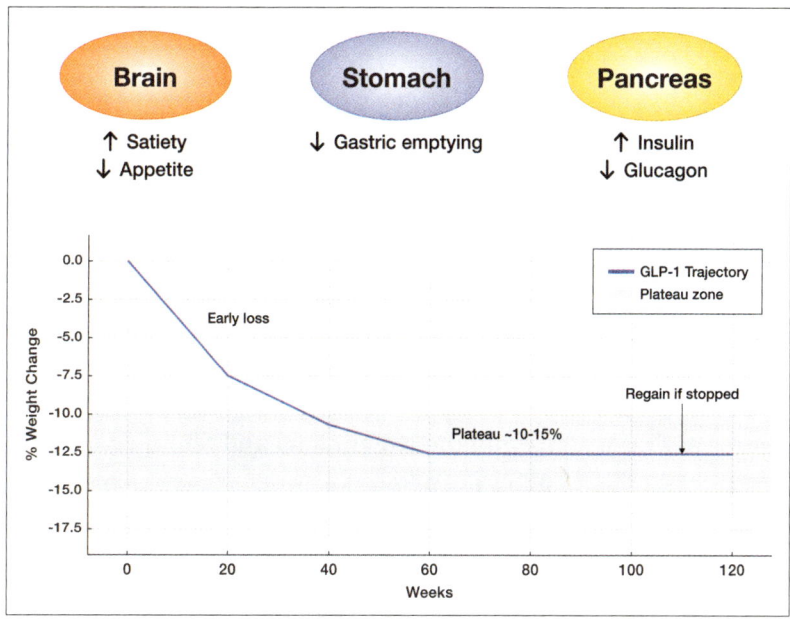

Figure 2. GLP-1 agonists act on the brain (increase satiety, reduce appetite), stomach (slow gastric emptying), and pancreas (increase insulin, reduce glucagon). The typical weight-loss curve shows an early drop, a plateau at around 10–15 percent of weight change, and weight can be regained if treatment stops

Then there are the side effects. Many people on these meds experience stomach trouble at first. Nausea is the most common—sometimes waves of it. It's so common that patients often say you have to "ride out the nausea" until your body adjusts. Vomiting, diarrhea, constipation, and bloating are also frequent complaints. There's even a new slang term, "Ozempic face," to describe the gaunt look caused by rapid weight loss, making wrinkles more pronounced. Your jeans feel looser, but your cheeks file a complaint. Rarely, more serious issues appear, such as stomach paralysis (gastroparesis), a condition that causes food to linger too long. In fact, surgeons now advise stopping these meds before any procedure with anesthesia, since a full stomach can lead to aspiration—food coming back up into your airways.

We also see occasional cases of pancreatitis (inflammation of the pancreas) and gallstones. Oh, and one more thing: Some users report mood changes and a kind of "flat" feeling emotionally. Sure, food isn't as appealing, but neither is much else. It's as if blunting the reward of eating spills over into an overall "meh" feeling. Not everyone experiences this, but it's something to watch out for.

If your goal is to see quick results on the scale, these shots might still tempt you. But ask yourself, "What's my long game?" Fast results impress the mirror; smart habits impress your future self. If it's sustainable weight loss and feeling good long term, you'll need a plan for when the "magic" of GLP-1s wears off. In fact, you might wonder, "Is there a natural way to tap into those appetite-taming, metabolism-boosting benefits without paying $1,000 a month or enduring a queasy stomach?" Good news: Your body has some weight-loss tricks up its sleeve. Next, we'll meet a surprising resident of your gut—one that could become your best weight-loss ally.

Meet Your Gut's Secret Weight-Loss Ally

If only you had a built-in appetite whisperer that didn't charge $1,000 a month... Spoiler: you do! Deep in your gut lives an army of microbes—bacteria, yeasts, and more—collectively called your gut microbiome. One little bacterial species in particular has been making a big splash in research for its link to healthy weight: *Akkermansia muciniphila*—let's call it Akker for short.

> 📌 **Gut Concept:** *Akkermansia*
>
> - **Full name:** *Akkermansia muciniphila*
> - **Nickname:** Akker (think of it as the mucus gardener of your gut)
> - **What it is:** A keystone gut bacterium discovered in 2004; an oxygen-intolerant microbe thriving in the mucus lining your intestines.

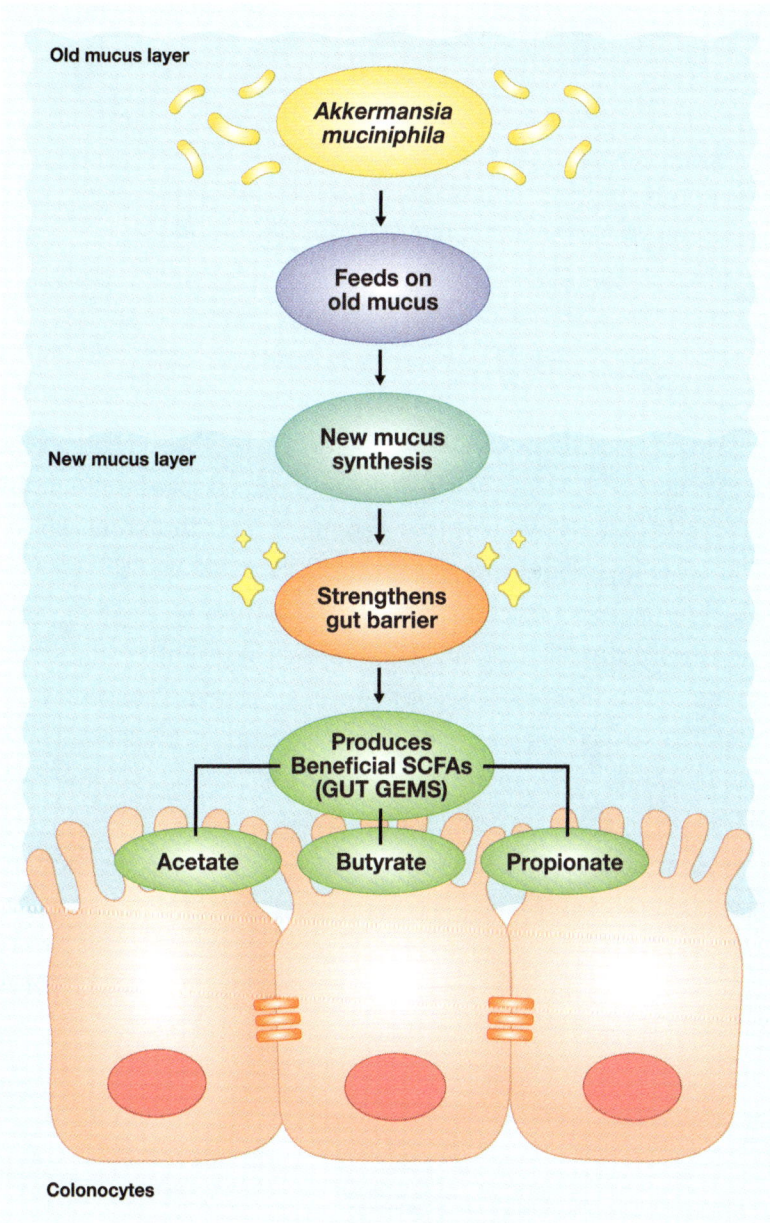

Figure 3. Akkermansia muciniphila *at the mucus layer: supports barrier renewal and produces SCFAs or "Gut Gems," mainly acetate and propionate*

- **Why *Akkermansia* matters:** By "tending" your mucus layer, Akker strengthens the gut barrier, supports other beneficial microbes, and produces short-chain fatty acids (SCFAs)—referred to as Gut Gems in this book—such as acetate and propionate; people with more Akker tend to be leaner, more insulin-sensitive, and less inflamed.
- **Big picture:** Akker is the quiet caretaker of your inner garden—keeping the protective mucus fresh and strong so your gut ecosystem can thrive.

Akker was discovered by scientists in the Netherlands. They managed to grow this shy microbe in a lab dish by feeding it exactly what it loves: mucus. Yes, the same slimy, protective layer that lines your gut. Akker hangs out right on your gut lining, munching away. Now before you say "Eww," this is actually a win-win. Here's how: By nibbling the older mucus, Akker stimulates your gut to produce fresh mucus—much like pruning a plant encourages it to grow back healthier. A thicker mucus layer means a stronger gut barrier and less irritation.

As Akker enjoys its mucus buffet, it produces helpful by-products, technically known as short-chain fatty acids (SCFAs). SCFAs are acids in the chemical sense, not the harsh, corrosive kind the word might make you think of. For clarity, we'll call them "Gut Gems." These Gut Gems are treasures your microbes make for you: They help nurture other beneficial bacteria, calm inflammation, and even boost your metabolism.

📌 Gut Concept: Gut Gems

- **Full name:** Short-chain fatty acids, mainly acetate, propionate, and butyrate
- **Nickname:** Gut Gems (the treasures that beneficial gut microbes produce)

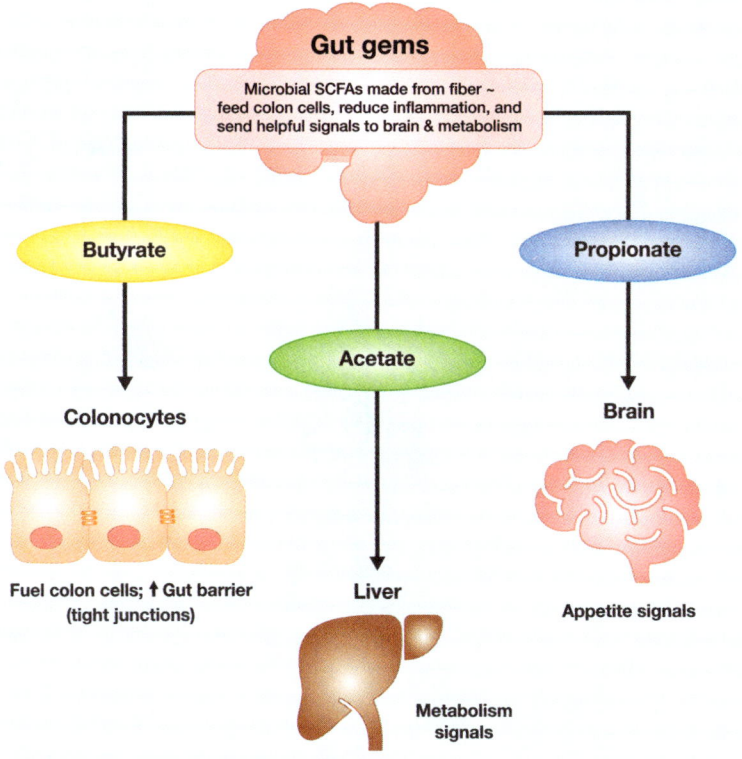

Figure 4. Microbial SCFAs fuel colon cells and signal metabolism and appetite.

- **What Gut Gems are:** Tiny fatty acids created when certain gut bacteria ferment fiber; they're the main fuel source for your colon cells.
- **Why it matters:** Gut Gems lower inflammation, seal and strengthen the gut barrier, regulate appetite hormones, and even rev up metabolism; butyrate in particular helps calm immune overreactions and support healthy energy production.
- **Big picture:** Gut Gems are the priceless currency of your gut economy, turning fiber into fuel and fortifying your defenses from the inside out.

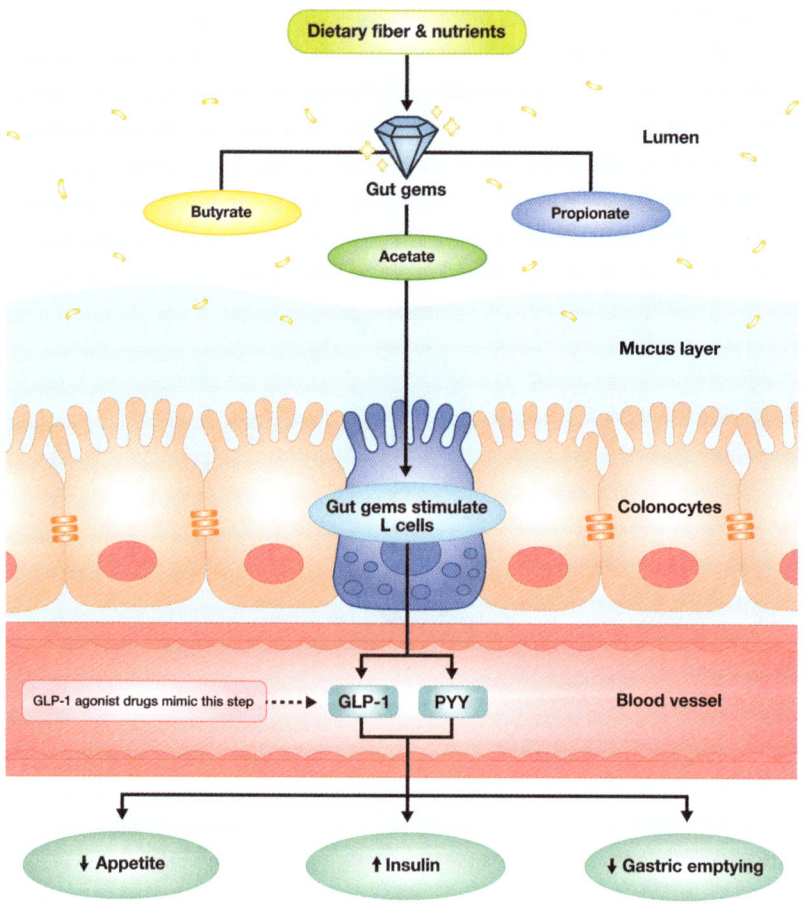

Figure 5. Gut Gems and nutrients nudge L cells to release GLP-1 and PYY, slowing stomach emptying and reducing appetite.

Researchers noticed something fascinating: Mice with lots of Akker stayed skinnier, even on a fatty diet; while those without it got fatter and developed insulin resistance, a precursor to diabetes. In humans, higher Akker levels have been linked to healthier weight, better blood sugar control, and less belly fat. While correlation doesn't necessarily prove causation, these findings suggest that having more of this bug goes hand in hand with better health.

Sure enough, a small human study found that taking Akker (especially the pasteurized form) for a few months, without other changes to diet and activity level, improved insulin sensitivity and lowered some cholesterol markers. It turns out that Akker's key components—the proteins it makes—can still interact with your gut even when the bacterium isn't alive. It still sends beneficial signals to your body that strengthen your gut and optimize metabolism. (Why it matters: Better insulin sensitivity means your body handles carbs and blood sugar more smoothly, which helps prevent energy crashes and belly-fat storage.)

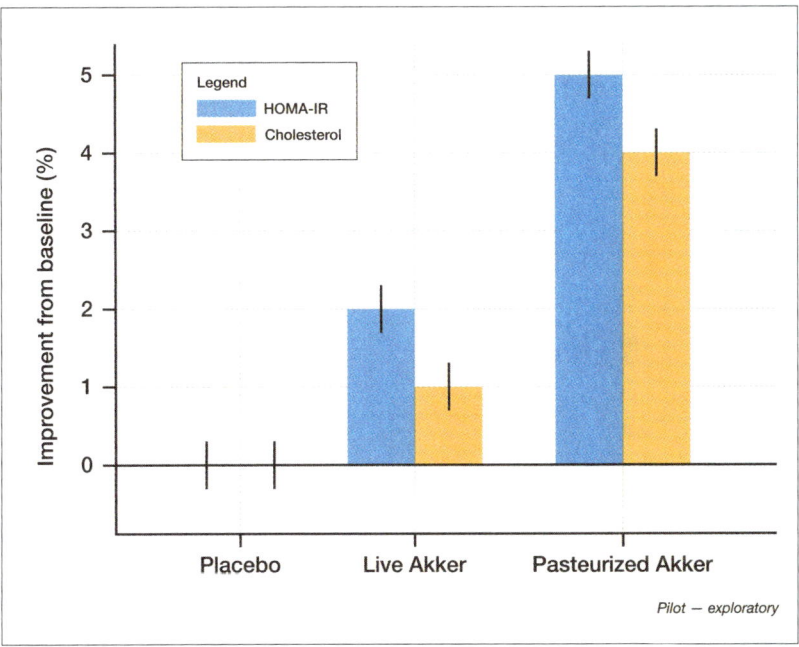

Figure 6. In a small pilot trial, pasteurized Akker improved insulin sensitivity (measured by Homeostatic Model Assessment of Insulin Resistance, or HOMA-IR) and cholesterol compared with placebo or live Akker. HOMA-IR is a lab score doctors use to check how hard your body is working to control blood sugar.

But before you rush to buy Akker supplements, keep in mind that it's not a magic bullet. Think of it more like a friendly mechanic tuning up your gut environment. It works best in synergy with a healthy diet. After all, this bug needs the right fuel, such as certain fibers and polyphenols, to thrive. In a healthy gut, Akker is beneficial. But some researchers caution that too much Akker could be harmful in a gut that's already inflamed or has a thin mucus layer. Balance is everything (more on that in the next sections).

The cool takeaway is that your own gut bacteria can become an ally in your weight-management regimen. By cell count, you have about as many microbial cells as human cells—so you might as well recruit some of them to your fitness team. Next, we'll explore how your gut sets the stage for these helpful bugs, and how a tiny detail such as oxygen makes all the difference.

Your Colon: A Low-Oxygen Paradise for Good Bugs

Ever wonder why gut bacteria, such as Akker, weren't discovered until recently? It's partly because they're absolute divas about their environment. They won't live just anywhere. Many of the best gut bacteria are what scientists call obligate anaerobes—a scientific way of saying they're oxygen-intolerant.

> **Gut Concept: Oxygen-Intolerant Gut Microbes**
>
> - **Full name:** Obligate anaerobes
> - **Nickname:** Oxygen-intolerant gut microbes (microbes that thrive only when air is absent).
> - **What it is:** Beneficial gut bacteria that view oxygen as toxic; they can only live and grow in the low-oxygen environment of your colon.
> - **Why it matters:** These microbes drive many of the gut's most important jobs, from fermenting fiber into SCFAs (Gut Gems) to protecting against pathogens; without a low-oxygen haven, they struggle to survive.
> - **Big picture:** These are the delicate deep-sea divers of your microbiome that need an oxygen-free zone to keep your gut ecosystem balanced and strong.

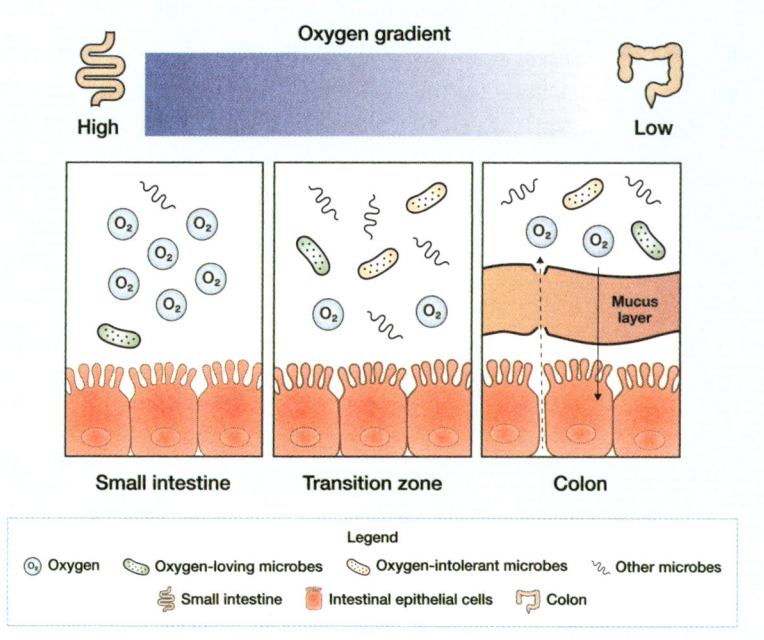

Figure 7. Oxygen gradient from small intestine to colon explains why anaerobes dominate the colon.

In the past, lab techniques weren't very good at keeping these oxygen-intolerant microbes alive, so entire communities of important gut bugs slipped under the radar. It wasn't until modern genetic tools came along (such as sequencing bacterial DNA directly from stool samples) that researchers realized what they'd been missing. It turns out the gut was teeming with these oxygen-intolerant critters quietly doing their work beyond the reach of old-school science.

Luckily your body provides the perfect home for these anaerobes. How it works: The deeper you go from the small intestine into the large intestine (colon), the less oxygen there is. Why? Because your own cells consume most of the oxygen. If your gut barrier is intact, very little diffuses back in. It's like walking from a bright, airy beach (your small intestine) into a dim, swampy marsh (your colon). That marshy colon environment is paradise for oxygen-intolerant microbes: They set up shop, ferment fiber, and throw a microbial party. However, when that barrier breaks down—a condition often called "leaky gut"—oxygen seeps in where it shouldn't be.

This matters because these organisms are the big fiber-eaters and nutrient factories in your body. Studies estimate that more than 90 percent of the bacterial species in your colon are these hard-to-culture, oxygen-intolerant bacteria. Besides signaling your brain and immune system to keep metabolism on an even keel, as previously discussed, they also produce vitamins and transform bile acids and other compounds into useful metabolites.

Keeping that low-oxygen zone intact is crucial. If too much oxygen sneaks into the colon environment (as a result of inflammation or leaky gut), it can tip the balance. Oxygen favors more "opportunist" bacteria—often those that don't contribute much to your health.

One key player in maintaining the zero-oxygen environment is your gut lining. Your lining cells gobble up oxygen as they work, keeping the neighborhood nice and oxygen-free. But if those cells get damaged or starved of their favorite fuel, they might not burn oxygen as effectively. Oxygen levels rise, and the balance shifts. The take-home message: Your colon is meant to be an almost air-free chamber where beneficial microbes flourish.

Fiber Fuel: How Good Bacteria Nourish Your Gut

Let's shine a light on those gut-lining cells we mentioned (the ones that help keep oxygen out). They're called colonocytes, and they are basically the brick and mortar of your colon lining. Guess what their favorite food is? Butyrate, a Gut Gem that your good bacteria make when they digest fiber. That's right—your gut cells and your gut microbes have a beautiful partnership, kind of like a farmer growing crops (fiber) to feed their livestock (bacteria), which then produce fertilizer (butyrate) to nourish the farm.

Here's how it works: You ingest fiber from an apple, and that fiber travels down to your colon mostly undigested by you—but your microbes have a feast. As they ferment the fiber, they release the Gut Gem butyrate. Colonocytes—the cells that line and support your colon—are the primary burners of this Gut Gem. They use this fuel to nourish your gut lining and, in the process, consume oxygen like crazy. This helps to create the perfect environment for oxygen-intolerant bacteria. These gut microbes are probably the most beneficial organisms in your entire body, and colonocytes make sure they have the pristine conditions they need to thrive. It's as if your gut cells are literally vacuuming up any stray oxygen, protecting the sanctuary of your microbiome.

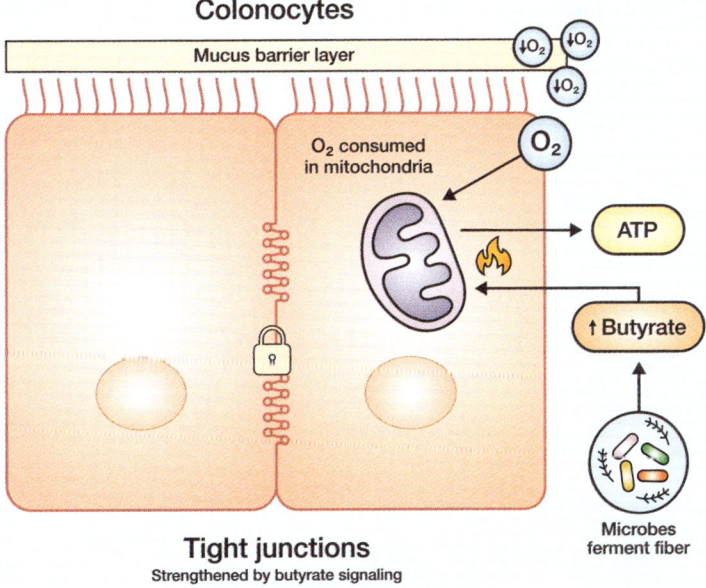

Figure 8. Butyrate fuels colonocytes, tightens junctions, and reinforces the mucus barrier.

Butyrate also acts as a signaler, telling those colon cells to fortify the gut. It encourages tighter connections between cells (imagine closing ranks so invaders can't slip through the cracks).

In scientific terms, butyrate upregulates proteins that form tight junctions, reducing "leaky gut." A strong gut barrier means toxins and bacteria stay in the intestines where they belong instead of sneaking into your bloodstream and causing inflammation.

Butyrate and friends (acetate and propionate) also coax your gut to produce more mucus and even antimicrobial peptides (natural antibiotics) that keep bad microbes in check. Beyond the gut, these Gut Gems send feel-good signals: Some travel to the liver and muscles to improve metabolism, while others chat with your brain to help control appetite and inflammation levels. In short, when your fiber intake is high and diverse, and you have a healthy microbiome to digest it, your gut bugs pump out a cocktail of chemicals that help your whole body function better.

Now flip the script: What happens on a low-fiber diet? Your poor colon cells don't get enough fuel. They start running on fumes, switching to less efficient energy sources such as amino acids—which means they burn less oxygen. The result is more oxygen lingering in the colon. Here's where it gets tricky. In someone with a healthy gut lining, low fiber is clearly a problem because it starves your good bugs.

But if your gut lining is already damaged and leaking oxygen inward, piling on fiber too early can make things worse. Pathogenic bacteria thrive in that oxygen-rich environment, gobble up the fiber, and crank out inflammatory toxins such as the endotoxin lipopolysaccharide (LPS), which radically impairs your immune system. In everyday terms, this means too much fiber, too soon, can backfire and feed the very microbes that cause gas, bloat, and inflammation. This is why a low-fiber diet can feel paradoxical—harmful in the long run, but sometimes therapeutic in the short term while you repair the gut barrier and restore balance.

When fiber is lacking, colon cells get less butyrate, causing the gut barrier to weaken and gaps to open between cells. It becomes a vicious cycle: Low fiber means less fuel for helpful microbes, which in turn creates a weaker gut barrier. Then, with more leakage, more inflammation occurs in the body.

This cycle can be broken simply by changing what's on your plate. Fiber may not make flashy diet headlines, but it's foundational—the steady fuel that powers the alliance between beneficial microbes and your colon cells.

We call this the fiber paradox: Fiber is your best friend once your gut is healed, but a potential enemy if you add it too soon. Think of it like watering a garden: If the soil is fertile, water makes everything grow beautifully. But if the ground is swampy and broken, adding more water just breeds weeds and rot.

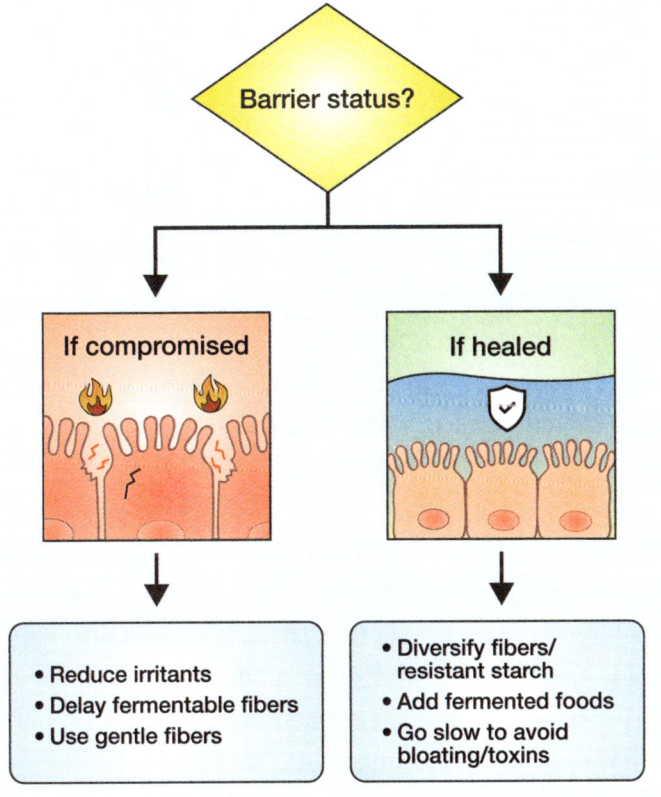

Figure 9. Add fermentable fibers only when the barrier is ready—go slow, then diversify.

When Modern Fats Attack the Gut

While we hear a lot about sugar and excess calories being bad for gut health, a less discussed culprit is the rise of industrial seed oils. These oils—such as soybean, corn, cottonseed, and safflower—are the cheap fats often used in fast-food fryers and packaged snacks. They're high in linoleic acid (LA), an omega-6 fat that is essential in small amounts; but in the massive quantities found in modern diets, it throws things out of whack.

> 📌 **Gut Concept: LA**
>
> - **Full name:** Linoleic acid
> - **Nickname:** Fragile fat (our shorthand for how easily this omega-6 fat breaks down into harmful by-products).
> - **What it is:** An omega-6 polyunsaturated fat (PUFS) found in seed oils such as soybean, corn, sunflower, safflower, and canola.
> - **Why it matters:** While tiny amounts are essential, the modern diet is drowning in LA. Because it's a fragile fat, it oxidizes easily, creating toxic aldehydes such as 4-hydroxynonenal (4-HNE) that can damage cell membranes, injure the gut lining, and fuel inflammation.
> - **Big picture:** Think of LA as a fat that spoils under pressure. Keeping it low and swapping in stable fats—butter, ghee, coconut oil, or tallow—helps protect your gut and overall health.

So, what's the issue? It comes down to chemistry. Fragile fats are polyunsaturated, meaning they have multiple double bonds. When we fry foods in these oils or leave them on the shelf too long, they break down and form oxidation products—rancid, toxic little molecules. One example is 4-HNE, a toxic compound that can wreak havoc in our bodies.

In the gut, these oxidized by-products can injure the cells lining your colon. Remember how butyrate is the preferred fuel? 4-HNE and its cousins can interfere with your colon cells'

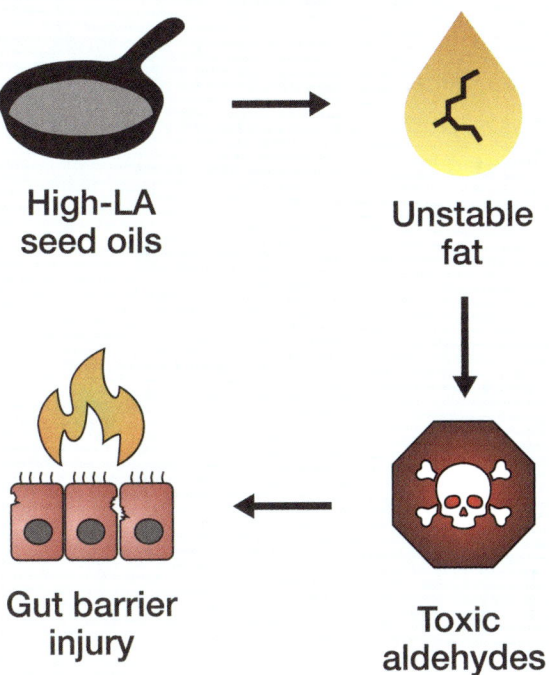

Figure 10. High-LA seed oils → lipid oxidation → 4-HNE → barrier damage and inflammation

ability to use butyrate by disrupting the mitochondria—the structures that produce energy. As a result, your colon cells burn less oxygen—and as we know, extra oxygen is the enemy of oxygen-intolerant bacteria.

Moreover, some of these toxic fat fragments can weaken the bonds between gut-lining cells. Think of your gut barrier as a tightly woven mesh: Oxidized oils stretch and tear holes in the fabric, allowing inflammation-causing particles to slip into the bloodstream.

Of course, seed oils aren't the sole villain here. Obesity and metabolic issues have many causes. Excess fructose (a type of sugar), overall calorie intake, and low activity are also big contributors. Lack of sleep is another important factor. But seed oils are a sneaky factor that have flown under the radar for a long time. In the last century, our intake of these oils has skyrocketed. We swapped butter for margarine and traditional fats for "vegetable" oils, thinking they were healthier. As seed-oil consumption climbed in the past decades, obesity rates also surged. While that doesn't necessarily prove a correlation, it's clear that something in our modern diet—beyond excess calories and insufficient exercise—is amplifying our weight struggles.

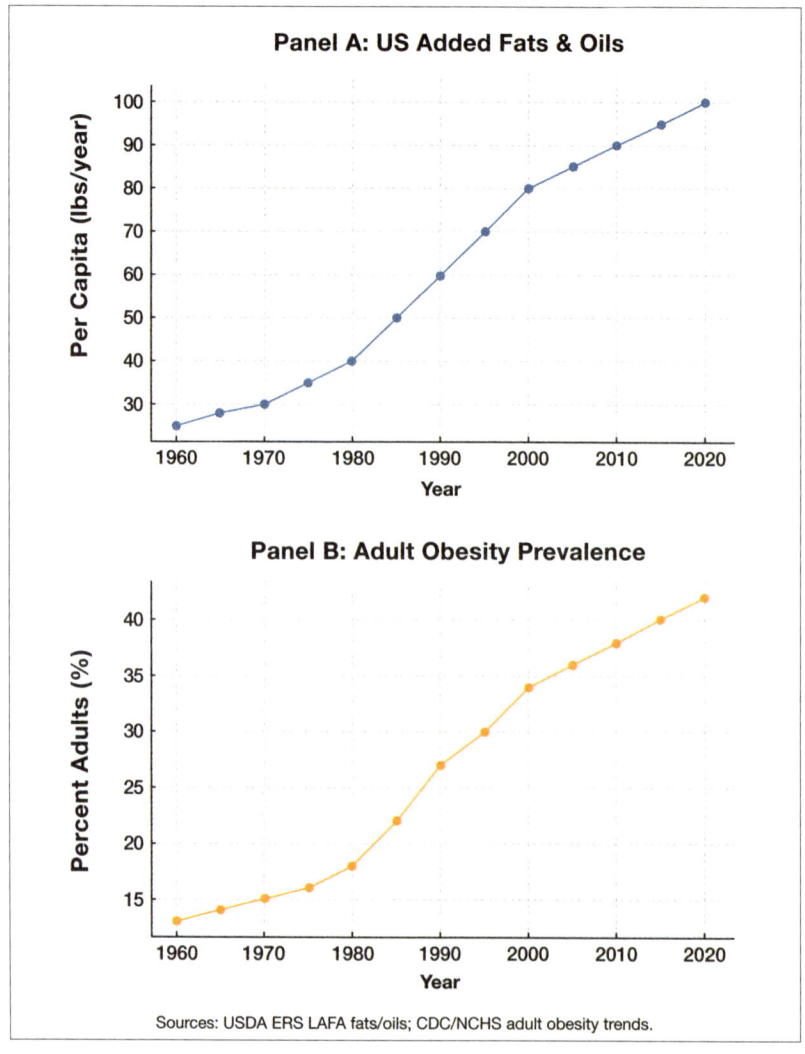

Figure 11. National data show parallel trends—but correlation isn't causation.

The practical tip here is to moderate your intake of these oils. It's okay to occasionally eat fries or other foods cooked in vegetable oil, but consider some swaps for day-to-day cooking. Traditional fats such as ghee, butter, or coconut oil don't produce as many nasty by-products. And of course, eating fewer deep-fried or ultra-processed foods in general will automatically cut down your exposure. The key point: The fats we choose can either support or sabotage our gut barrier and microbiome.

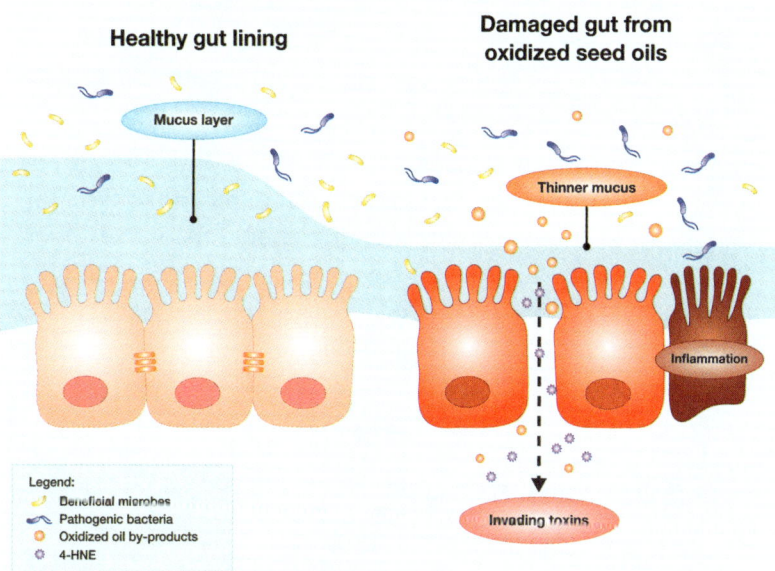

Figure 12. Oxidized seed oils thin the mucus layer and generate toxic by-products (e.g., 4-HNE), weakening the barrier and fueling inflammation.

Microbe Magic: The GLP-1 Boost from Your Belly

Remember that GLP-1 hormone we talked about—the one those weight-loss shots mimic? Well, your gut can ramp up GLP-1 on its own under the right circumstances, no medication needed. The L cells in your small intestine—especially the ileum—and your colon work as tiny hormone factories that sense when food is present and release GLP-1 along with other appetite-related hormones.

📌 Gut Concept: GLP-1

- **Full name:** Glucagon-like peptide-1
- **Why the name?** Looks structurally like glucagon, a different hormone, but has very different effects.
- **What it does:** Released after meals, especially when carbohydrates or fat hit the small intestine; slows stomach emptying, enhances insulin release, suppresses glucagon (which otherwise raises blood sugar), and reduces appetite.
- **Big picture:** GLP-1 is your gut's "metabolic conductor," keeping blood sugar in check while telling your brain you've had enough food. It's also the natural pathway today's weight-loss drugs try to mimic.

Another key player is peptide YY (PYY). (The "YY" comes from the two tyrosine amino acids at the tail end of the molecule.) What matters more than the chemistry is the effect: PYY is a satiety hormone. After you eat—especially if your meal is rich in protein and fat—your L cells release PYY into the bloodstream, sending a signal to your brain that you're full. PYY works with GLP-1 to curb appetite and steady digestion.

Gut Concept: PYY

- **Full name:** Peptide YY
- **Why "YY"?** Two tyrosine (Y) amino acids at its tail.
- **What it does:** Released after eating; slows gut movement and signals your brain that you're full.
- **Big picture:** PYY is your gut's built-in portion controller, teaming up with GLP-1 to help you stop eating when your body has had enough.

Now, our microbial buddy Akker has a neat trick: It produces certain proteins that appear to stimulate the L cells to secrete GLP-1. Two of these proteins, P9 and Amuc_1100, interact with the gut in ways that appear to boost GLP-1 release. Think of them as Akker's little "buttons" that press your gut's appetite-control switch.

📌 Gut Concept: Amuc_1100

- **Full name:** Amuc_1100 (a protein found on the surface of *Akkermansia muciniphila*).
- **Nickname:** Akker's Key (one of the main ways Akker unlocks health benefits in your body).
- **What it is:** A cell-surface protein produced by Akker; even when the bacterium is dead, this protein can still interact with your gut lining and immune system.
- **Why it matters:** Binds to receptors on your intestinal cells, strengthening the mucus barrier, calming inflammation, and helping to regulate metabolism; this is why pasteurized (heat-killed) Akker can still deliver health benefits—it preserves the protein.
- **Big picture:** Amuc_1100 is Akker's signature handshake with your body, a tiny protein with big influence, proving you don't always need live bacteria to see powerful effects.

This microbial magic might be nature's way of balancing intake. You feel fuller sooner and longer, just as you would with the medication—but since it's a natural process, you experience far fewer side effects.

Now, to be clear, this boost is subtler than what you'd see with a synthetic injectable drug. You won't drop twenty pounds in a month just by boosting Akker. But over time, a healthier microbiome can help regulate appetite and cravings. Some people taking Akker supplements or eating diets that increase Akker report they snack less and feel more in control of their portions—findings that early studies suggest may be linked to Akker's effects.

There's also growing interest in whether Akker's GLP-1 boost can improve blood sugar control. Early signs are promising. In one small trial, those given Akker showed better fasting glucose and lower insulin levels. Essentially it's improving metabolism, just as the drugs do, but from the inside out.

One day we might even see a head-to-head face-off: Akker versus Ozempic. We're not there yet, but there's encouraging evidence that Akker may offer many of the same benefits as GLP-1 injections. And here's another twist: You might not even need live bacteria to tap into these effects. That's where postbiotics come in.

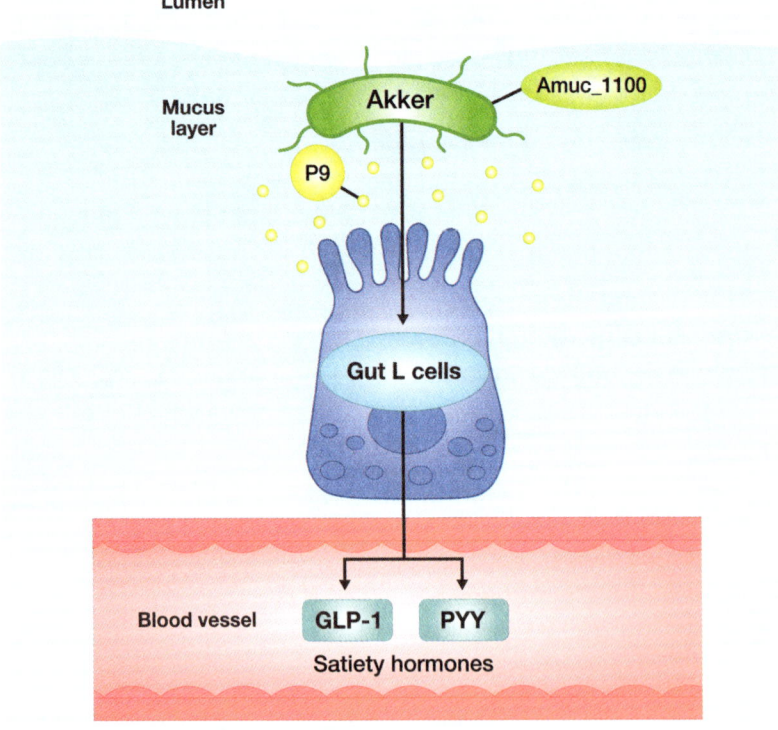

Figure 13. L cells release GLP-1 and PYY; Akkermansia proteins (P9/Amuc_1100) nudge secretion.

Dead or Alive: Bacterial Benefits Either Way

While it may sound counterintuitive, even dead bacteria can deliver benefits. Researchers have coined a term for the nonliving products of beneficial microbes: postbiotics. It's a bit like how vaccines work—using inactivated germs, or parts of them, to train your body. In the gut, postbiotics rely on the "remains" of good bugs to prompt healthy changes.

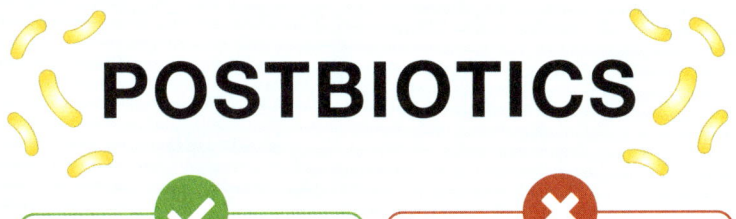

Figure 14. Postbiotics are preparations of inanimate microbes/components with demonstrated benefits.

Postbiotics can be made up of inactivated bacterial cells, fragments of their cell walls, or purified compounds they produce—such as specific fatty acids, enzymes, or vitamins. The key is that these substances can interact with your body's cells and receptors to trigger healthy responses. Even a dead bacterium may hold the key to unlocking a beneficial pathway.

Akker is a prime example. Scientists found that pasteurizing (heat-killing) Akker didn't remove its positive effects. In fact, in some studies it actually worked better. Why? One theory is that, without the chance to grow too much or behave unpredictably, the dead Akker is all benefit and no risk. Its cell wall contains unique proteins (such as Amuc_1100, dubbed "Akker's Key") that remain after pasteurization. These proteins can interact with receptors on your intestinal and immune cells, instructing them to "strengthen the gut lining here" or "make more of that GLP-1 hormone."

Another advantage of postbiotics is their safety and stability. Live probiotics must survive manufacturing and packaging—not to mention the trip through your stomach's harsh environment. Postbiotics, like purified proteins or bacterial preparations, are generally more shelf-stable. There's also virtually no risk of unintended colonization.

We're still in the early days of postbiotic research, but small trials look promising. Apart from Akker, other postbiotics have shown benefits in calming inflammation, boosting immune responses, and reducing symptoms of irritable bowel syndrome (IBS). Postbiotics are essentially probiotics in a more controlled, predictable package.

This might mean that in the near future, your doctor or dietitian could recommend a specific postbiotic supplement—say, a capsule of Akker proteins—targeted to your specific needs (weight loss, blood sugar control, gut healing, etc.). A-Mansia Biotech in Belgium, for example, has already commercialized a pasteurized form of Akker following its approval as a novel food in the European Union, and others are on the horizon.

That said, whether we're discussing prebiotics (fiber), probiotics (live bugs), or postbiotics (beneficial bug parts), the endgame is the same: improving the gut environment. In short, postbiotics allow us to hack our biology safely—and you'll likely hear more about them as research races ahead. Now, if you do opt for live probiotics—especially Akker—how do you make sure they reach your colon alive? Let's tackle that real-life challenge next.

Getting Probiotics Past the Harsh Gauntlet

You see all those labels bragging about "50 billion CFUs" in probiotics? That number means nothing if the bacteria don't survive the trip. Thinking of popping a probiotic pill to get these benefits? The fact is, hardly any of these oxygen-intolerant bacteria survive the journey from your mouth to your colon. First of all, with a pH around 1 or 2, your stomach acid kills most bacteria—good or bad—on contact. The bacteria that manage to survive the acid will next have to make it past the bile in the small intestine. Bile is a harsh fat detergent that can puncture bacterial membranes.

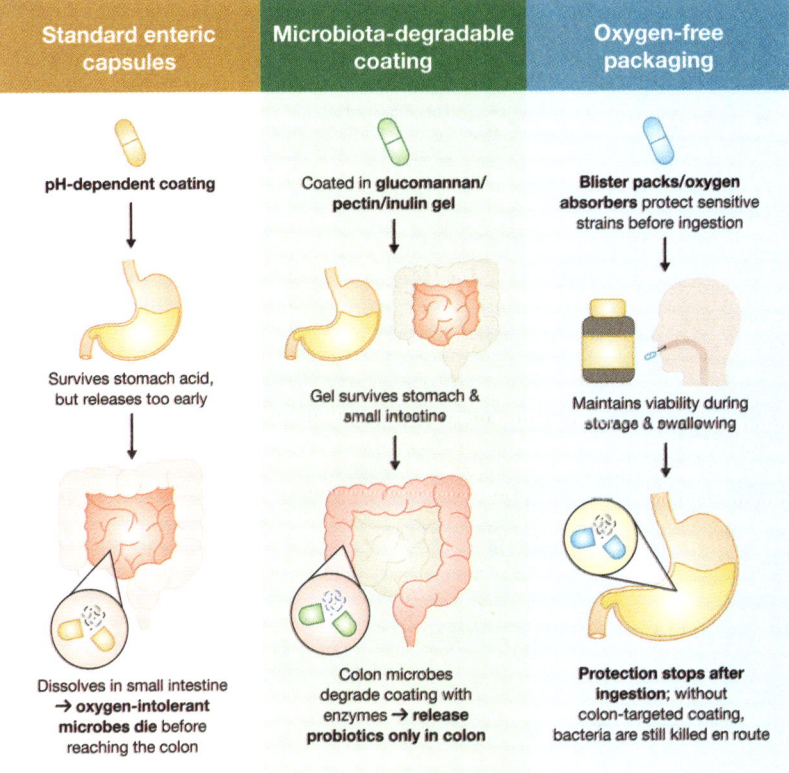

Figure 15. Targeted coatings and oxygen-safe packaging matter more than headline CFUs.

Next up are powerful digestive enzymes such as trypsin and chymotrypsin—their day job is to chop proteins into their constituent amino acids—that can also damage delicate probiotic cells. Why it matters: These enzymes can shred delicate probiotics before they ever reach your colon. Finally, there's oxygen—we already know what that does to these bacteria. Of course, exposure to oxygen is almost inevitable during manufacturing and storage.

In short, by the time you swallow probiotics, the sensitive ones may already be dead or will die in transit down your gut. So how do we give these good bugs a fighting chance? Give them armor and a map!

Scientists and supplement makers are developing protective delivery systems:

- **Enteric-coated capsules:** These have a special coating that resists stomach acid and dissolves only when the pH is higher (such as in the small intestine). That way the bacteria aren't released into the acidic pool of the stomach but instead in a safer environment further along.

- **Microcapsules and beads:** Some probiotics are put into tiny alginate beads or polymer coatings meant to act like armor, surviving stomach acid and dissolving later in the intestines. The problem is that, like standard enteric capsules, these coatings usually dissolve long before reaching the colon—the very place oxygen-intolerant microbes need to live. By the time the capsule breaks down, most of the bacteria are already dead and never make it to their final destination.

- **Oxygen-free packaging:** High-quality probiotics sometimes come in blister packs with oxygen absorbers to keep them dry and air-free until swallowed. But while packaging protects them on the shelf, it offers no defense once inside your body. Without true colon-targeted delivery, most microbes are wiped out before they arrive in the colon.

- **Novel "synbio" coatings:** Coating bacteria in a fiber gel–like glucomannan (from konjac root) is a clever targeted delivery trick. Your stomach and small intestine can't digest it, but colon microbes can—so they break down the gel and release the probiotics right where they're needed.

> 📌 **Gut Concept: Colon-Targeted Delivery**
>
> - **What it is:** Colon-targeted delivery is a probiotic system that uses a glucomannan fiber coating (from konjac root).
> - **Why it matters:** Unlike enteric capsules or polymer beads that may dissolve too early, glucomannan is an indigestible polysaccharide in the human digestive tract. It stays intact until it reaches the colon, where microbial enzymes called mannanases can finally break it down.
> - **Big picture:** This means the capsule could take twenty minutes or twenty hours to pass through your digestive tract, but it will only open in the colon, right where oxygen-intolerant microbes such as Akker need to be. Colon targeted delivery is one of the most reliable ways to ensure nearly all of the bacteria survive and reach their true home.
>
> **Bottom line:** If you buy a probiotic for gut health, choose one with proven colon-targeted delivery. Even the best probiotic needs right packaging to survive the trip—and fiber once it arrives.

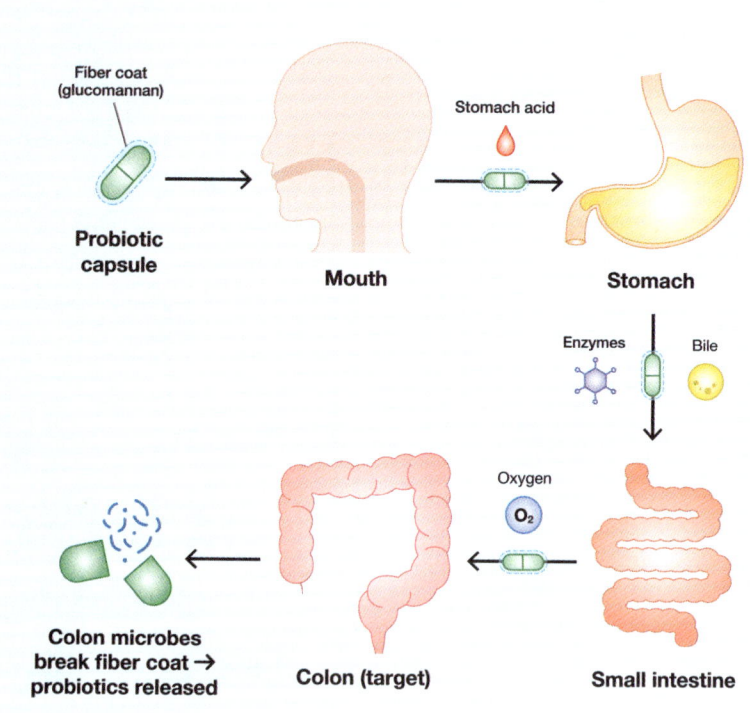

Figure 16. The probiotic gauntlet—acid, bile, enzymes, oxygen— and colon-targeted glucomannan as a solution

Fiber: The Unsung Hero in Your Weight Journey

We've sung fiber's praises quite a bit so far—but what exactly is it? Dietary fiber isn't just one thing; it's a whole family of plant carbohydrates that your body can't fully digest but your gut microbes love. Different types of fiber do different things, so variety is key.

Broadly, fiber falls into two camps: soluble and insoluble. Soluble fiber—found in foods such as oats, beans, apples, and flaxseeds—dissolves in water and forms a gel. This gel slows digestion and feeds the bacteria in your colon, leading to lots of Gut Gem production. Insoluble fiber—think wheat bran, veggie peels, nuts—doesn't dissolve; it adds bulk to stool and helps keep things moving, which can help prevent constipation.

Then there's resistant starch, a special kind of carb that acts like fiber. It's found in cooked-and-cooled potatoes or rice (ever heard that day-old cold rice is healthier?), green bananas, and legumes. Resistant starch is a favorite fuel for butyrate-producing bacteria—it can lead to a big butyrate boost in your colon.

> 📌 **Gut Concept: Resistant Starch**
>
> - **What it is:** Resistant starch is a type of starch that "resists" digestion in your stomach and small intestine, passing through untouched until it reaches the colon.
> - **Why it matters:** Because your enzymes can't break it down, resistant starch becomes food for your gut microbes. When they ferment it, they produce Gut Gems such as butyrate, which helps strengthen your gut lining, reduce inflammation, and even improve insulin sensitivity.

Type	Food Examples	Main Effects
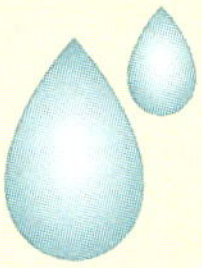 Soluble fiber	Oats, beans, apples, flaxseeds	• Forms gel in gut and it slows digestion & prolongs fullness • Gentle rise in blood sugar • Fermented by gut bacteria that produces lots of SCFAs
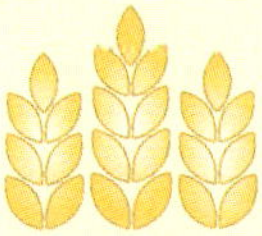 Insoluble fiber	Wheat bran, veggie peels, nuts	• Adds stool bulk • Speeds gut transit • Helps prevent constipation
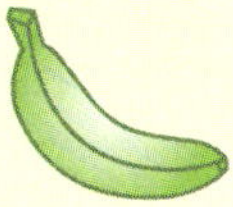 Resistant starch	Cooled cooked potatoes or rice, green bananas, legumes	• Acts like fiber • Fuels butyrate-producing bacteria • Boosts colon butyrate levels that increases gut health benefits

Figure 17. Soluble versus insoluble fiber and resistant starch, with simple food examples and effects

- **Where to find it:** It is common in foods such as green bananas, cooked-and-cooled potatoes or rice, legumes, and oats.
- **Big picture:** Resistant starch is like a care package that skips digestion and lands directly in your colon, nourishing the oxygen-intolerant microbes that keep your gut ecosystem thriving.

Reality Check

If you've been eating a low-fiber diet with lots of refined flour, high-fructose corn syrup, and processed foods, suddenly downing huge amounts of fiber can shock your system. You might get gas, bloating, or even an upset stomach. In an unhealthy gut (inflamed or "leaky"), an overload of fermentable fiber can feed the wrong bacteria and produce excess toxins such as LPS (a bacterial toxin that, as mentioned, triggers inflammation). Think of it like starting a workout routine: You don't go from the couch to sprinting a 5K in one day without some pain.

Start low and go slow. Add an extra serving of a fiber-rich food each day—for example, swap whole-grain bread for white bread—and see how you feel. The next week, introduce beans or lentils. Gradually your gut microbes will adapt and flourish without overwhelming your system.

And don't forget to hydrate! Staying hydrated will help prevent discomfort as you increase fiber. Also consider adding polyphenols to your high-fiber meals. These feel-good microbes found in berries, tea, coffee, and olives are great at taming inflammation.

A fiber-rich diet isn't about boring bran cereal—it's a rainbow of whole foods: fruits, veggies, whole grains, nuts, seeds, and legumes. Flavor them with delicious herbs and spices (more polyphenols!). Be creative in adapting them to your own preferences. For example, start your day with oatmeal topped with berries and nuts, enjoy a hearty bean-and-veggie soup for lunch, snack on an apple with peanut butter, and cook quinoa, roasted broccoli, and grilled chicken for dinner. High-fiber eating can be flavorful and filling. Your gut will respond with steadier energy, better digestion, and easier weight control.

The Two-Phase Plan to Repair and Rebuild

Now let's put everything together into a road map for harnessing your gut to support weight loss—and overall health. Think of it in two phases: (1) Repair your gut environment (fix the soil). (2) Reseed it (plant the garden).

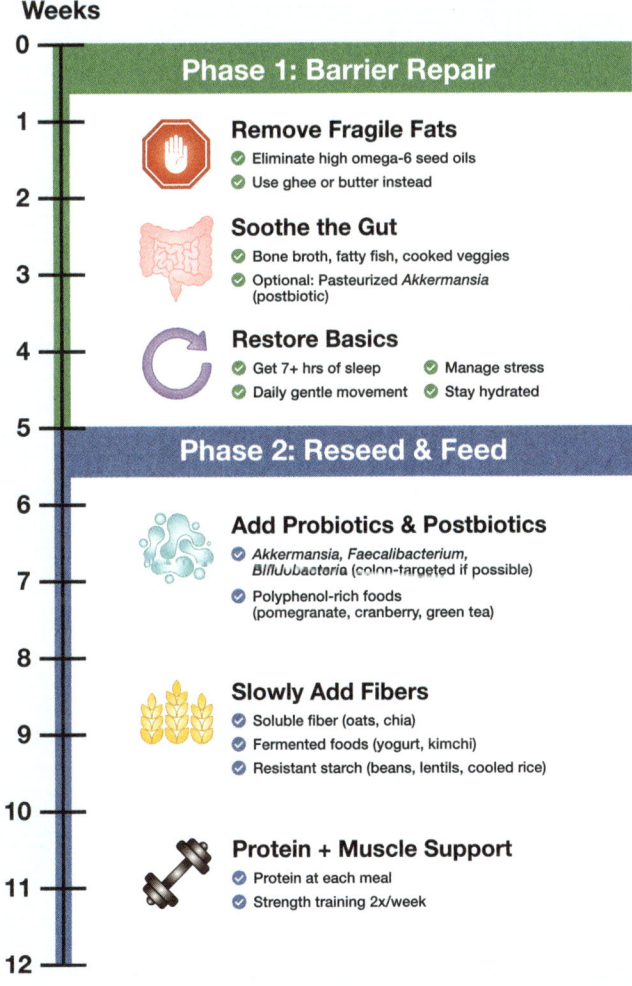

Figure 18. Two-phase gut plan: phase 1 (barrier repair) → phase 2 (reseed and feed)

Phase 1: Barrier Repair (Weeks 0–4)

For the first month, focus on healing your gut lining and removing irritants:

- **Ditch the bad fats.** Reduce the chemical irritation in your gut by cutting out high omega-6 seed oils and swapping in butter, ghee, tallow, or coconut oil for cooking. Skip the deep-fried foods (sorry, fries!), at least for now.

- **Soothe your gut.** Fortify the mucus layer and calm inflammation by adding a pasteurized Akker (postbiotic) supplement, if available. If not, include gut-friendly foods such as bone broth (rich in gut-healing nutrients), fatty fish (anti-inflammatory omega-3s), and cooked veggies (easy fiber and polyphenols).

- **Practice lifestyle basics.** Prioritize sleep (aim for seven to eight hours, since your gut repairs itself at night). Manage stress—try walks, meditation, or anything that relaxes you. Move your body gently each day (exercise boosts blood flow and digestive function). Finally, stay hydrated (your gut cells need water to rebuild effectively).

By the end of phase 1, you should notice less bloating, improvements in skin and mood, and possibly a couple of pounds lost just from cutting out the junk and calming inflammation. More importantly, you've set the stage for the next phase.

Phase 2: Reseed and Feed (Weeks 5–12)

With your gut on the mend, you can now populate it with beneficial microbes:

- **Reintroduce good bugs.** Add a quality probiotic now if you can, especially one with Akker, *Faecalibacterium*, or friendly *Bifidobacteria* strains. Make sure it's enteric-coated or otherwise protected. No Akker supplement available? Support your own Akker production by eating foods rich in polyphenols such as cranberries, pomegranates, or unsweetened green tea.

- **Continue the healing aids.** Keep up any postbiotic supplement or gut-friendly foods from phase 1. Consistency is key.
- **Gradually increase fiber.** Each week, introduce one new fiber-rich food. For example, start with oatmeal or chia seeds (soluble fiber) one week, add beans or lentils the next (resistant starch and fiber), and finally add a fermented food such as yogurt or kimchi (bonus microbes). The goal is to feed your new microbial buddies without overwhelming your system. Go slow and pay attention to your body's signals.
- **Focus on protein and strength.** To ensure you're losing fat and not muscle, include protein at every meal (eggs, Greek yogurt, lean meats—whatever you prefer). Do a bit of strength training a couple of times a week (even bodyweight exercises at home will work). More muscle means a higher metabolism and helps prevent the "skinny-fat" or "Ozempic face" look from muscle loss.

Keep tuning in to your body as you progress. If your energy is rising and cravings are fading, you're on the right track. If something causes bloating or discomfort, pull back and reintroduce it later. Around the three-month mark, you may find you've shed weight steadily, your blood sugar and cholesterol have improved, and your appetite feels more under control. These changes aren't just about the scale—they set you up for better overall health, slashing your risk for type 2 diabetes, heart disease, and even some cancers linked to obesity.

Even if you decide to use a GLP-1 medication at some point, you'll have built a solid foundation of habits. That will make any treatment more effective and help prevent weight regain if you stop the drug. Who knows—you might realize you don't need the shot now that you've addressed the root causes.

Bottom line: This isn't an overnight miracle but a long-term fix that actually works.

Weight-Loss Conquests: Your Victory Checkpoint

Today's 3-point scorecard:

1. **Change oil:** Replace one cooking oil or processed snack with a healthier fat option today.

2. **Find fiber:** Add one new fiber-rich food—such as a cup of veggies or a spoonful of flaxseed—to feed your good gut bugs.

3. **Move and rest:** Take a brisk fifteen-minute walk and aim for a full night's sleep—simple steps that boost your gut and mood.

Claim your badge and remember that big changes start with small steps—every healthy choice counts!

CHAPTER 2

GLP-1 Drugs: A Consumer-Friendly Blueprint

Imagine this: You've been on a new weight-loss shot for six months and the results are miraculous. Your jeans are loose, coworkers are showering you with compliments, and the scale shows numbers you haven't seen in years. You feel like you've discovered the holy grail of weight loss.

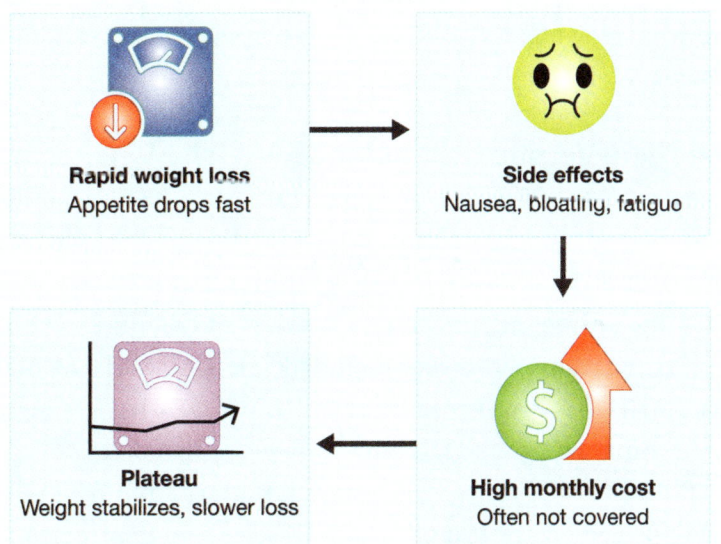

Figure 19. Real-world GLP-1 journey: rapid early loss → side effects → cost → plateau

Each week you've given yourself a tiny jab of Ozempic. In the first few weeks, you had to remind yourself to eat, and the pounds flew off faster than you could buy smaller clothes. On the other hand, you are living on saltine crackers and ginger tea to soothe the nagging nausea.

Then there's the fact that this "miracle" is burning a huge hole in your wallet. Insurance might cover it if you had diabetes or severe obesity, but you're taking it mostly to slim down. So, you pay hundreds of dollars a month out of pocket and wince each time you refill.

Emotionally it's a roller coaster. Food used to be a joy—pizza night with family, your mom's cookies; now it barely interests you. At times your mood feels oddly muted, as if someone turned the dial down on your day-to-day excitement.

And now the kicker: After six months of glory, the weight loss has stalled. In fact, a couple of pounds crept back on when you skipped a dose during a stomach bug. So, what now? It's time to get real about what these drugs actually do, how long they work, and what side effects to expect. In other words, here's what the ads won't tell you.

The Hype Versus the Evidence

If you've spent five minutes on social media, you've no doubt encountered the hype around GLP-1 drugs like Ozempic, Wegovy, and Mounjaro. Hailed as "skinny shots" by Hollywood stars and online influencers, the marketing machine—both the official drug ads and the unofficial TikTok testimonials—makes it sound like these injections turn off hunger like a light switch. You'd think we'd found the cure for obesity in a pen.

But what does the evidence say? First, a reality check: GLP-1 agonists are medications originally developed to treat type 2 diabetes. As we discussed in the last chapter, they mimic a hormone your gut naturally makes when you eat, signaling your pancreas to release insulin and your brain to register fullness.

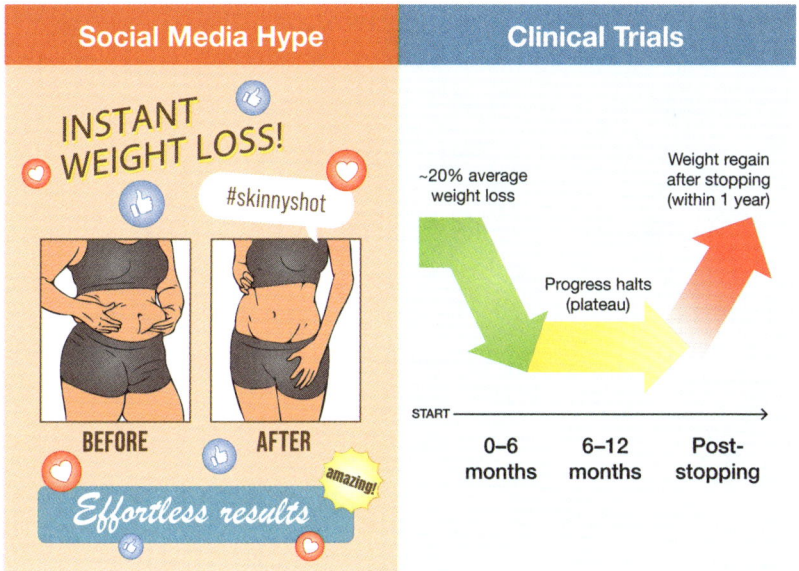

Figure 20. Hype versus data: what trials show versus social media claims about GLP-1 agonists

In clinical trials for obesity, many people lost about 15 percent of their body weight over a year—significantly more than with diet and exercise alone.

That's solid evidence that these drugs can work—within limits. That's the catch: within limits. These injections aren't fairy dust that will cause fifty pounds to melt away with no effort. They work best in people who have a lot of weight to lose or specific conditions such as diabetes or a BMI over 30. They're FDA-approved for type 2 diabetes and chronic weight management in people with obesity (or overweight with weight-related health issues)—that's it. Using them as a quick fix to drop a dress size for summer or to counteract too many desserts is venturing into off-label territory. Yet the hype has everyday people with a few pounds to lose clamoring for a prescription their doctor might not even agree to write.

Yes, GLP-1 drugs can help you lose weight, sometimes dramatically. But they don't turn you into a superhuman who can eat anything you want and stay skinny forever. The evidence shows you'll lose weight only as long as you keep taking the medication. While marketers paint a picture of quick, effortless weight loss, in reality you'll still need to do some work to get the full benefit.

What They Actually Do to Your Body

Let's get down to the nitty-gritty: What exactly is happening inside you when you're on a GLP-1 drug? In short, your digestion slows way down and your hunger cues get tampered with. On a GLP-1 agonist, food you ate hours ago might still be in your stomach. This delayed gastric emptying is exactly the point: If food stays put longer, you feel full and stop eating more. Great for portion control! But the flip side is that when food sits too long in your stomach, it can lead to nausea, bloating, or acid reflux. This is a big reason people on GLP-1 medications often experience that heavy, sluggish stomach feeling.

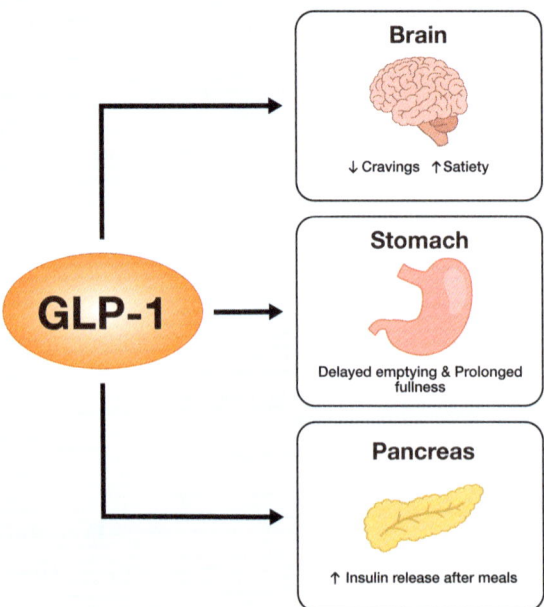

Figure 21. GLP-1 slows gastric emptying and reduces appetite; brain satiety circuits stay engaged longer than normal.

Slowing down digestion has another consequence: It can affect medical procedures that require an empty stomach. If you need anesthesia, that food in your belly becomes a risk. Anesthesia and a full stomach are a dangerous mix because inhaling food into your lungs is a potentially serious complication. That's why many anesthesiologists now recommend pausing GLP-1 drugs days in advance of any procedure, just to be safe.

These meds also tweak your metabolism. They prompt your pancreas to release more insulin when you eat and signal your liver to release less sugar, keeping blood sugar steadier. They also act on your brain's appetite-control center to dial down cravings. The exact mechanism involved here is still being studied, but it's possible the drug is influencing reward circuits in the brain.

Durability Problem: Watch That Weight Creep Back

So, you've been riding the weight-loss express thanks to a GLP-1 drug—fantastic! But as soon as you stop the medication, the magic stops and your appetite roars back to life like a lion that's been caged too long. The numbers on the scale start to creep up again. This isn't the permanent fix you thought it was.

One major study found that participants who stopped taking semaglutide (sold under the brand names Ozempic and Wegovy) after a year regained roughly two-thirds of the weight they had lost within the next year. Think about that—if you dropped thirty pounds on the drug, you're likely to regain around twenty pounds once you're off it. You didn't do anything wrong—it's biology in action. The medication was suppressing your appetite. Once it's gone, your body pushes back. Hunger hormones such as ghrelin (the one that makes your stomach growl) ramp back. Your now lighter body also burns fewer calories at rest than when you were heavier. In short, your system *wants* to regain weight, and without the drug's help, it often succeeds.

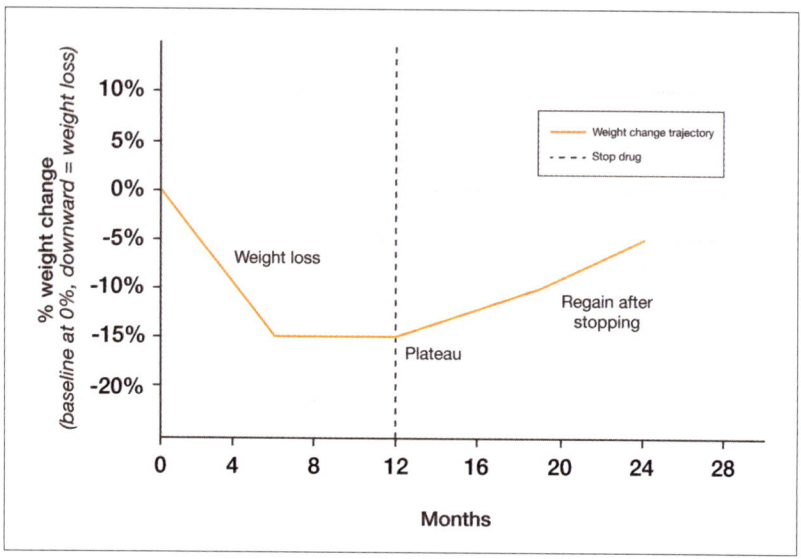

Figure 22. After stopping semaglutide, approximately two-thirds of lost weight returns within one year.

This means if you want to keep the weight off, you either have to stay on the medication indefinitely or have a rock-solid maintenance plan—or ideally both. And "indefinitely" is a daunting prospect, financially and health-wise. Not only could that cost you tens of thousands of dollars over a lifetime but the long-term effects of these meds are still unknown. Doctors generally agree that obesity is a chronic condition, and treatments might be needed long-term, just like blood pressure pills or insulin. But many patients start these shots thinking they'll use them for a few months, hit their goal weight, and be done.

Another wrinkle: The weight loss from GLP-1 drugs can hit a plateau even while you're still injecting. Most people see rapid loss in the first three to six months, after which the pace slows. At that point, some people get tempted to increase the dose or, if they're already at the max, may feel discouraged. It's important to know that this leveling off is normal—your body likes equilibrium.

Bottom line: These medications are a tool, not a permanent cure. Keeping the weight off will require continuing the drug or using other strategies. The key is going in with eyes open: Plan for the long game, not just the first sprint.

Everyday Side Effects: Common but Explainable

Most side effects from GLP-1 drugs are mild, but almost everyone experiences at least one. About three out of four users report some gastrointestinal effects. Here are the big ones:

- **Nausea:** About 50 percent feel at least a bit queasy. This often hits when you first start or when your dose increases. It usually improves as your body adjusts.

- **Diarrhea:** About 30 percent deal with occasional loose stools.

- **Vomiting:** About 20 percent experience vomiting, often when they've eaten a bit too much or too quickly on that slow-to-empty stomach.

- **Constipation:** About 10–15 percent experience the opposite problem—things slow down too much, causing infrequent bowel movements.

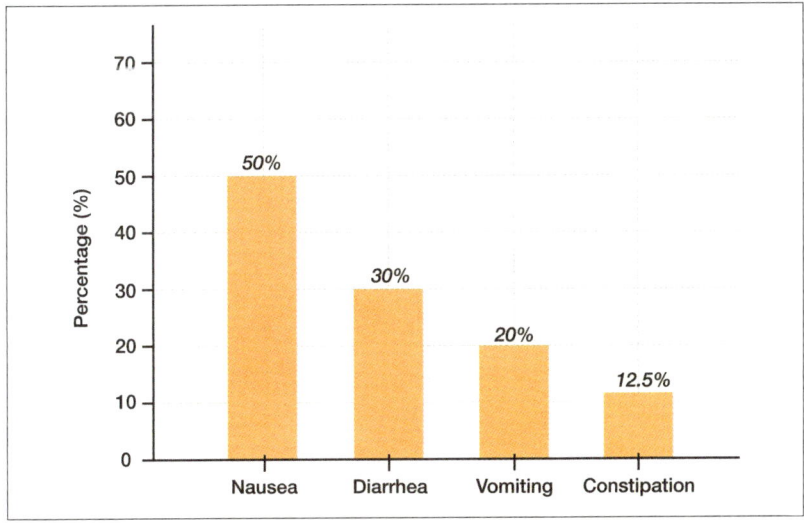

Figure 23. Common GI effects—nausea, diarrhea, constipation—stem from delayed emptying.

Then there's the famous "Ozempic face." Actually, this hollowed-out look can happen with any rapid weight loss, not just these drugs. Roughly 8 percent of users notice it. The good news: It usually improves once your weight stabilizes.

It's normal to feel a bit lousy in the beginning: mild nausea, an occasional bout of vomiting or loose stool, or constipation. Serious alarms are rare. If you can't keep any fluids down (risking dehydration), if you're vomiting everything you eat for more than a day, or if you have severe belly pain that doesn't go away, it's time to call your doctor. They might tweak your dose or give you something for nausea if needed. Also, no bowel movement at all for many days combined with pain is a red flag.

Serious Gut Risks: When Digestion Slows (Gastroparesis) or Stops (Ileus)

We've covered the garden-variety stomach issues, but there are some rarer, more serious digestive problems to know about. At the forefront is gastroparesis, or partial stomach paralysis. Think airport security at peak hour—everything lines up, nothing moves. There's some evidence that GLP-1 drugs can cause gastroparesis in susceptible individuals. One recent study found between seven and ten in one thousand patients on a GLP-1 drug ended up with a gastroparesis diagnosis. Essentially the drug's effect of slowing stomach-emptying goes too far in some people. Typically once the medication is stopped, the stomach will gradually return to normal, but not always overnight. A few unlucky people have had symptoms persist for a long time, even after coming off the drug.

Another related issue is ileus, which is paralysis of the intestines that can lead to blockage. Think of it as the conveyer belt in your gut grinding to a halt. If nothing moves, you can imagine the discomfort: severe bloating, pain, and vomiting. Ileus is very rare on these medications, but there have been reports of bowel obstruction. An ileus or obstruction is an emergency, period.

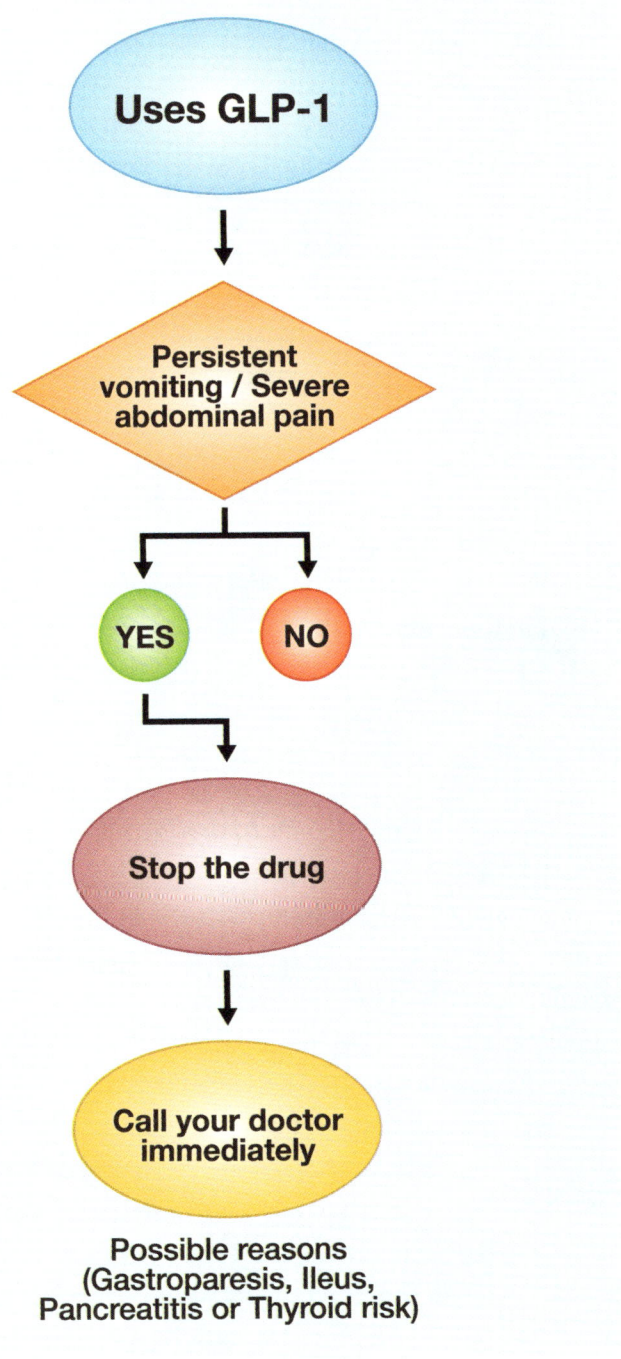

Figure 24. Rare but serious: Gastroparesis/Ileus—know red-flag symptoms.

We also need to talk about pancreatitis, or inflammation of the pancreas, which can cause severe abdominal pain (often radiating to the back) and vomiting, and can land you in the hospital. Some early reports linked GLP-1 drugs to pancreatitis, but the data is mixed. Some large studies didn't find a big difference, while a few analyses did find a slight uptick in pancreatitis cases. One analysis suggested the risk might be severalfold higher in people using GLP-1s for weight loss. If you have a history of pancreatitis, these drugs should be used with caution and close medical supervision. If you're on one and get sudden, unrelenting upper belly pain with vomiting, get it checked out right away.

Lastly, let's mention the thyroid. In rodent studies, high doses of GLP-1 drugs caused a specific thyroid tumor called medullary thyroid carcinoma (MTC). This hasn't been seen in humans at normal doses, but it's a signal worth noting. If you have a personal or family history of this rare thyroid cancer, or the genetic condition multiple endocrine neoplasia type 2 (MEN2), these meds are a no-go.

Gallbladder and Biliary Alarms

Dropping a lot of weight quickly can have another uncommon but real side effect: gallstones. This was true long before GLP-1 drugs—crash diets and bariatric surgery often trigger gallstones—and the condition is showing up with these meds, too. Why does rapid weight loss cause gallstones? Your gallbladder stores bile, which helps digest fat. If you're eating much less fat, your gallbladder isn't emptying as regularly. Bile can sit and become sludgy, and cholesterol in the bile can crystallize into stones. Basically your gallbladder acts like kitchen staff for fat; cut orders too sharply and the staff takes an unscheduled break. So, keep the line moving: small, regular meals help the "kitchen" stay open. Rapid weight loss also shifts the balance of substances in bile, making stone formation more likely.

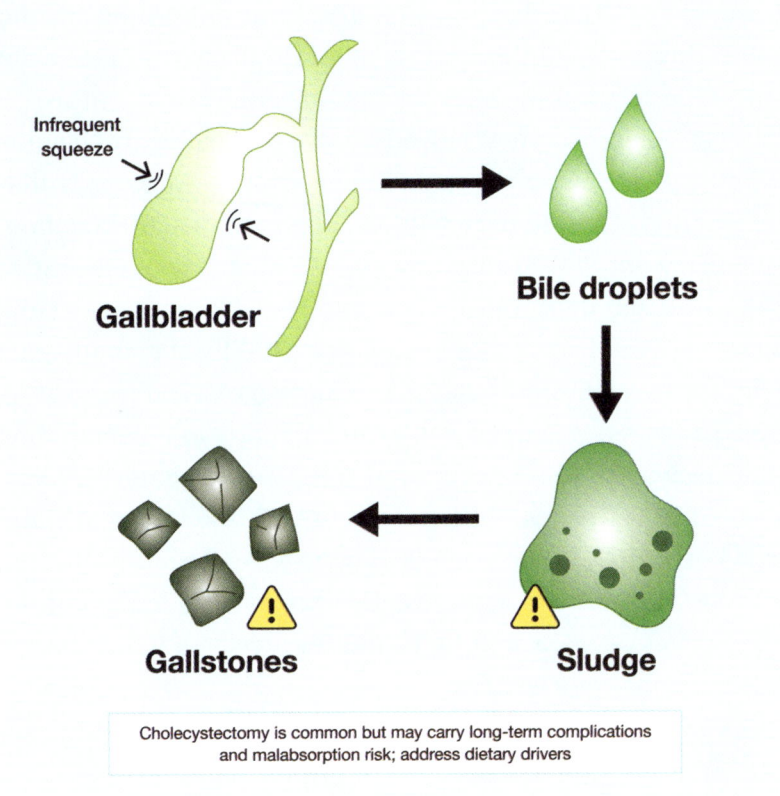

Figure 25. Rapid weight loss increases gallstone risk.

Studies confirm that GLP-1 users have a higher chance of gallbladder and bile duct issues than nonusers. The risk is still fairly low, but it's elevated. If you get a sharp pain under your right rib cage that doesn't go away—especially if you feel nauseous or notice yellowing in your eyes—get checked out by a doctor as soon as you can. To lower your risk, try to stay hydrated and don't skip meals entirely. And remember that slower, steadier weight loss is gentler on your gallbladder than a rapid drop.

Eyes on the Signal: Vision Risks

When we think about the risks of weight-loss drugs, we don't usually consider our eyesight. It's not exactly an expected connection: Take a shot to lose weight, risk going blind? While vision-threatening side effects from GLP-1 drugs are rare, some concerning signals have doctors paying attention.

That concern has now moved into the courtroom. Thousands of patients are suing the makers of Ozempic, Wegovy, Trulicity, Mounjaro, and Rybelsus in ongoing multidistrict litigation. Among the alleged harms: gastrointestinal injuries such as gastroparesis and ileus, blood clots, and vision loss. The lawsuits accuse drugmakers Novo Nordisk and Eli Lilly of downplaying or failing to warn about such risks while aggressively marketing their products. Litigation has also expanded to compounding pharmacies accused of selling unapproved or counterfeit versions of GLP-1 drugs. With case counts in the thousands and growing in 2025, serious complications have become part of the broader conversation about whether the safety profile of these blockbuster drugs was fully communicated to patients before prescriptions were written.

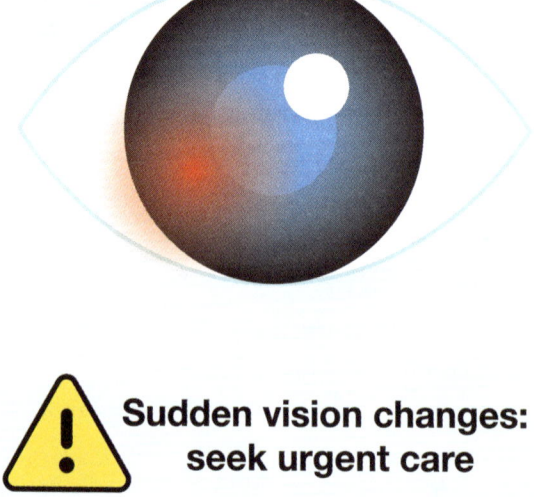

Figure 26. Rare signals: Monitor for sudden vision changes.

One of the rare eye conditions that has popped up is nonarteritic anterior ischemic optic neuropathy (NAION)—quite the mouthful. In simpler terms, NAION is an eye stroke: Blood flow to the optic nerve gets cut off, causing sudden, often permanent vision loss in one eye. Usually NAION occurs randomly or in people with cardiovascular risk factors (and sometimes with certain medications for erectile dysfunction). Now a handful of case reports have noted NAION happening in patients on GLP-1 drugs. A recent review tallied around nine instances of serious vision problems that might be linked to these meds, including NAION, optic nerve inflammation (papillitis), and maculopathy (retinal damage).

If you have diabetes, you probably already know about diabetic retinopathy, an eye disease in which high blood sugar damages the retinal blood vessels and threatens vision. What's surprising is that rapid blood sugar improvements, such as when starting a GLP-1 drug, can sometimes make retinopathy temporarily worse. It's a paradox: Better sugar control helps eyes long-term, but the quick change can exacerbate existing eye problems in the short term. In fact, in one semaglutide diabetes trial, more people on the drug had retinopathy progression than those on a placebo, presumably for this reason. So, if a diabetic patient has retinopathy, doctors need to monitor their eyes closely when starting these drugs. The takeaway for you: If you're on a GLP-1 and experience any vision changes—blurriness, partial vision loss, or anything unusual—treat it seriously and seek medical attention.

Muscle and Bone: What You Lose Along the Way

Let's shift to a sneaky consequence of weight loss itself. When you lose weight, it's not only fat that disappears. Our bodies can be a bit indiscriminate when calories are cut and will burn muscle tissue along with fat. In addition, hormonal changes during weight loss can lead to a loss of bone density. This loss of what's called "lean mass" can happen whether your weight loss occurred through dieting, surgery, or medications such as GLP-1 agonists.

In the context of GLP-1 drugs, roughly 15 percent to 30 percent (or even more) of weight lost may be lean mass rather than fat. Why does this happen? When you eat a lot less, and if you're not keeping up protein intake and staying active, your body can start breaking down muscle for energy. Carrying less weight means your bones have less loading, which over time can cause loss of bone density, similar to how astronauts lose bone density in low gravity.

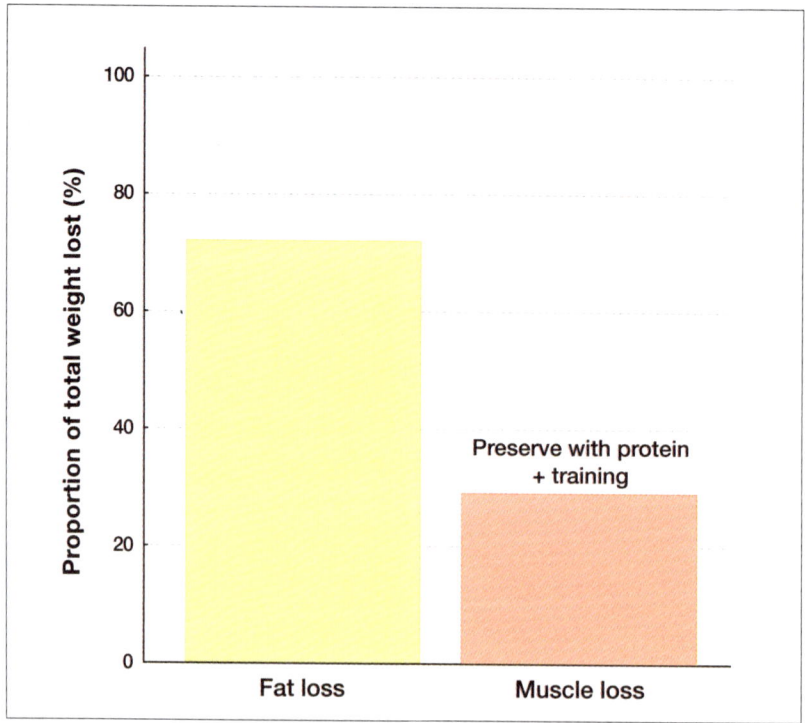

Figure 27. Protect lean mass: 15–30 percent of loss may be lean tissue.

Losing muscle might not sound like a big deal when you're focused on the scale, but it *is* important for your long-term health and keeping the weight off. Muscle is your metabolic engine, burning calories even at rest. If you lose a lot of muscle, your metabolism slows, and you might find it easier to regain weight. Plus, muscle strength is key to staying mobile and independent as you age. Bone loss is quieter but also matters. Weaker bones mean higher fracture risk down the line.

The strategy for fighting this muscle and bone loss is simple: protein and pumping iron. Proteins are the building blocks of muscle—make sure you're eating enough of it. And do some form of resistance exercise—lifting weights, bodyweight exercises, resistance bands—two to three times a week. This will help you retain muscle mass and even strengthen bones. There are tools that allow you to track your body composition over time (through scans or measurements). But at the very least, pay attention to your strength and energy. If you notice you're feeling weaker or more fatigued, that's a cue to up the protein and adjust your exercise routine. Remember, the goal isn't just a smaller number on the scale; it's a healthier, fitter you. So celebrate fat loss but also make sure you're protecting your lean mass.

Surgery and Procedures: Aspiration 101

We touched on this earlier, but it's worth a reminder: Anesthesia and a non-empty stomach can be a dangerous combo because of the risk of breathing in stomach contents (aspiration). If you're on a GLP-1 drug and you need surgery or sedation, let your medical team know. The standard presurgery fasting rules might not be enough for you.

Many anesthesiologists now have guidelines for patients on GLP-1 drugs. So if you're going in for anything—even a colonoscopy—mention your weight-loss medication. Your doctors will give you specific instructions regarding if and when to pause it.

All this is to say that the slow-gastric-emptying effect of GLP-1 drugs is more than just a quirky side effect; it has real implications for your safety in certain scenarios. With proper

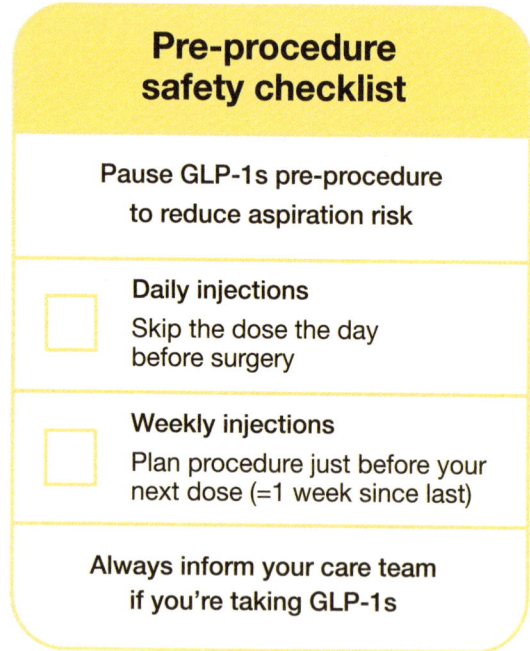

Figure 28. Pause GLP-1s pre-procedure to reduce aspiration risk.

planning and pausing the med as directed before procedures, you can avoid Aspiration 101 from ever being more than a theoretical concern.

Mental Health Signals: What We Know—and Don't

An aspect of GLP-1 drugs that's just starting to get attention is their effect on your mental health and mood. Along with diminished "food noise" or cravings, some users have reported emotional blunting—as though life's volume knob got turned down a notch. For some people, less interest in food becomes a feeling of less joy or interest in life generally.

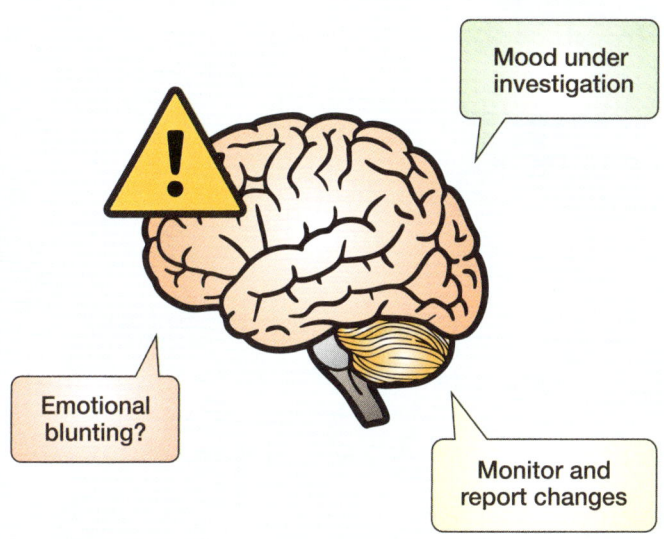

Figure 29. Mood signals under investigation—monitor for emotional blunting.

Regulatory agencies in Europe are investigating these medications for possible links to suicidal ideation, but there's no definitive evidence as of yet. The clinical trials for these drugs didn't show a spike in suicide or major mood disorders compared to placebo, but vigilance and further research are warranted given case reports and pharmacovigilance signals, especially in patients with preexisting psychiatric conditions.

The scattered cases and personal stories mean we can't completely dismiss it. We know these drugs act on the brain's pathways to reduce cravings and possibly affect dopamine, so it's plausible there could be psychological effects for some people.

What should you do? Keep an eye on your mood. If you start feeling consistently down or having dark thoughts you normally wouldn't, tell your doctor right away. Don't ignore your mental health. Losing weight isn't worth it if it takes away your peace of mind.

Costs, Coverage, and Counterfeit Problems

We've talked biology, now let's talk budget. As we're well aware, GLP-1 drugs come with a hefty price tag. A month's supply of semaglutide can easily run near or above $1,000 out of pocket. Mounjaro (tirzepatide) and others are similarly priced.

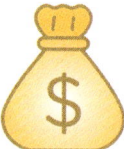

Costs
- Around $1,000 per month
- Adds up to thousands yearly
- Some savings programs exist

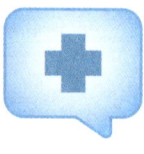

Coverage
- Usually covered for diabetes
- Rarely covered for weight loss
- Coverage varies by insurer/employer

Counterfeit
- Fake Ozempic pens reported
- Shady compounding/online sellers
- Risks: ineffective or unsafe drugs

Figure 30. Costs, coverage variability, and counterfeit risks

Many insurers draw a line at covering meds for weight loss, labeling treatments as "cosmetic" or nonessential. If you have type 2 diabetes or life-threatening obesity, insurance is more likely to cover something like Ozempic. As a result, many people wanting to lose weight with these injections end up facing a big out-of-pocket bill. Even if you can afford it for a short while, what about the long term? Needing it for a year or more could mean spending tens of thousands of dollars.

This high cost has spawned a wild west of unofficial options. Maybe you've seen the social media ads or gotten a tip about obtaining cheap semaglutide from compounding pharmacies. Beware: There's been a surge in counterfeit products, and the FDA has even warned that fake Ozempic pens have been found in the US supply chain. In search of a bargain, some have received a fake product that didn't work. Some people have even gotten sick from what they thought was a legitimate GLP-1. Compounding pharmacies can legally mix drugs under certain conditions, and not all of them are bad. But some offering "discount semaglutide" might be using unapproved raw ingredients or something entirely different.

Real-World Adherence and the Whiplash Effect

It's one thing to start a medication; it's another to stick with it. In the real world, people often take these GLP-1 drugs for a while, then stop (due to side effects, cost, or life events), and sometimes restart later. This on-and-off pattern can lead to a "whiplash" effect on your body and progress. Stopping suddenly can cause your appetite and cravings to come rushing back, and weight can rebound. If you restart later, those initial side effects might return because your body lost its tolerance. It can become a cycle: Lose weight on the drug, regain the weight when off of it. Yo-yoing like this isn't great for your body or morale.

In studies, about one in ten patients stopped early due to side effects. Outside of trial settings, more stop because of cost. Not staying on these meds long-term makes maintaining results harder.

So what can you do? Have a game plan. If you decide to pause or stop the medication, do it with your health-care provider's guidance and a strategy in place. Taper off slowly or ramp up

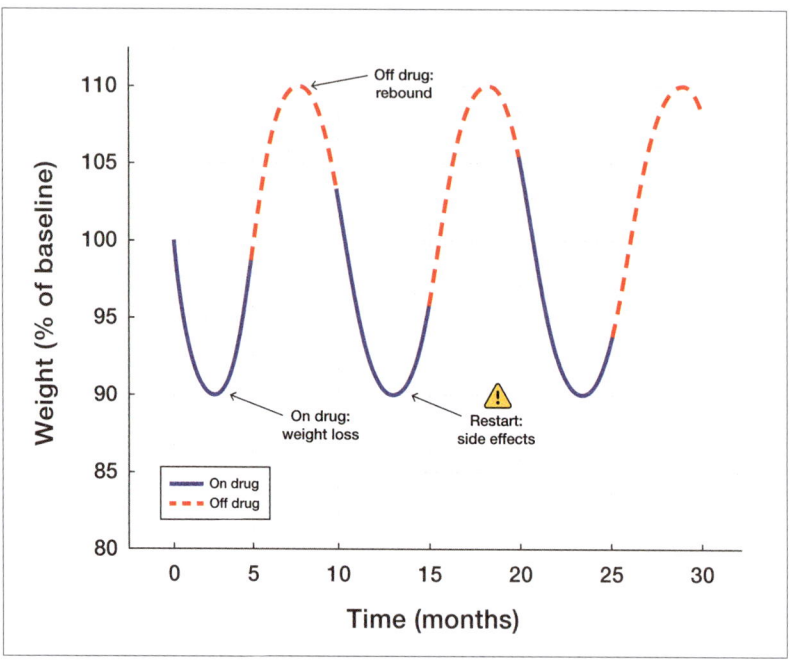

Figure 31. On-off use leads to rebound and side-effect reset.

your diet and exercise to compensate. Ideally avoid these drugs altogether. I believe pasteurized (postbiotic) Akker is a far better long-term strategy.

Remember, consistency is key in weight management. It's better to go slow and keep the weight off than to lose it fast and regain it even faster. Life will throw curveballs with vacations, family celebrations, holidays, and stress, but try to stay consistent with your plan, whether or not you're on medication. If you have to stop, do it purposefully and keep working on your health another way. The journey doesn't end just because you change tactics.

Smarter, Safer Paths Forward

After hearing about all these pros and cons, you might be wondering how to move forward in a sensible way.

GLP-1 Drugs: A Consumer-Friendly Blueprint

If you and your doctor decide to use a GLP-1 medication, then set yourself up for success and safety. Follow the dose schedule exactly; don't rush to a higher dose hoping for faster results, which can backfire with side effects. Treat the drug as scaffolding and keep building healthy habits around it. Prioritize protein in your meals and do resistance exercises a couple of times a week to preserve muscle and keep metabolism fired up. Stay on top of side effects and communicate with your health-care provider. In short, consider the medicine one tool in an arsenal of healthy weight strategies. Try to stay active, well nourished, and attentive to your body.

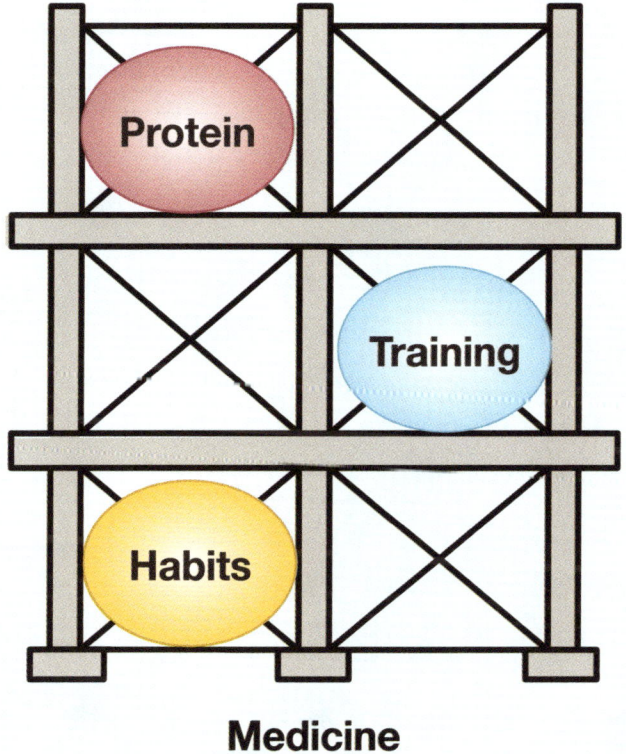

Figure 32. Medication as scaffolding: pair with protein, training, and healthy habits.

And don't go it alone. A strong support system—whether that's a nutritionist, a weight-loss program, or an app—can make all the difference in keeping you accountable and motivated. This is where the Mercola Health Coach app comes in. It's a technologically advanced, personalized guide built to adapt to your unique circumstances. The app not only helps you spot the excessive fragile fats in your diet—the biggest hidden driver of weight gain—but also serves as your exercise companion. It can accurately assess your current fitness level, then recommend and guide you through a customized training plan designed to preserve and build muscle. That's key, because maintaining lean mass is what will keep your weight under control in the long term.

To make it easy, we've created a QR code you can scan to download the Mercola Health Coach app for free. Think of it as your pocket coach—always ready to nudge you toward better food choices, smarter movement, and a more sustainable path to health.

Your Free Pocket Health Coach
Scan. Download. Start today.

Take the guesswork out of weight loss and fitness. The Mercola Health Coach app gives you:
- A personalized nutrition guide that identifies hidden fragile fats sabotaging your progress
- Smart fitness assessments with tailored exercise plans to protect your muscle and keep you moving
- Real-time coaching to keep you accountable and on track

 Scan this QR code to get FREE access to the Mercola Health Coach app. This tool allows you to log your meals, track your macronutrient ratios, and monitor your progress over time.

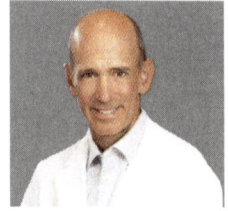

Informed Consent over Hype

GLP-1 weight-loss drugs aren't magic potions; they're powerful meds with real trade-offs. The key is to approach them with informed consent—understand what you're getting into. Think of this chapter as your crash course, so you can tune out the hype and make the decision that's right for you.

Here's a quick checklist of what to keep in mind if you're considering or using these drugs:

- **Common side effects:** Expect some nausea or stomach upset (especially early on).
- **Serious risks:** While unlikely, know the red flags for gallbladder issues, pancreatitis, and vision changes, and report anything severe to your doctor.
- **Body composition:** Not all weight loss is fat. Protect your muscle with protein and strength exercise so you lose the *right* weight.
- **Mental health:** Monitor your mood. If you feel unusually down or not yourself, speak up.
- **Procedures:** Always inform your doctors if you're on a GLP-1 before any surgery or medical procedure.
- **Costs and commitment:** Plan for the expense and how long you'll stay on treatment. Be prepared if coverage changes or if you need to stop.

There's no free lunch in weight loss—but with good information, you can plan a path to a healthier you. Stay curious and remember *you* are in the driver's seat of this journey.

Weight-Loss Conquests: Your Victory Checkpoint

Today's 3-point scorecard:

1. **Get strong.** Plan a strength-training session (or any resistance exercise) this week to help protect your muscle mass during weight loss.

2. **Check in.** Plan daily check-ins with yourself to observe your mood and energy levels.

3. **Move in the morning.** Create a morning habit with a form of exercise that you genuinely enjoy.

CHAPTER 3
The Origin Story of Akker

Remember our old friend Akker and how it wasn't discovered until 2004? Before we do a deep dive into its origin story, let's meet the first "hype man" for gut microbes: Élie Metchnikoff. Metchnikoff (1845–1916) grew up in Ukraine, studied zoology, and became fascinated with how organisms defend themselves against disease. His biggest breakthrough was discovering phagocytosis (white blood cells swallowing bacteria), which earned him the 1908 Nobel Prize in Physiology or Medicine. In his later years, he chased a different question: Why did some communities live longer? His answer was delightfully culinary: fermented milk. Metchnikoff's overarching claim—that longevity flows from the gut—foreshadows this book's thesis: By repairing the gut barrier, feeding it the right microbes, and keeping fragile fats in check, the need for drugs shrinks.

Observing that Bulgarian villagers who ate loads of yogurt and kefir often lived to advanced ages, Metchnikoff argued that lactic acid bacteria could crowd out microbes in the colon and reduce what he called autointoxication. He even drank sour milk daily, convinced it would extend life. The idea gained popularity via newspapers and ads, but the lab tools of the day were insufficient to prove this; most gut bacteria refused to grow on plates, so the science stalled even as the yogurt craze rolled on. After World War II, antibiotics stole the spotlight, and gut microbes were cast as villains. Yet in Japan and the Soviet bloc, the popularity of fermented-milk cultures with *Lactobacillus* and *Bifidobacterium* kept Metchnikoff's ember glowing.

Although the term *probiotic* only arrived in the 1950s and '60s, the core idea was already there. With antibiotics came the belief that medications were the cure for everything. Symptom relief, rather than root-cause repair, was the order of the day. (This is exactly the illusion we'll dismantle, one section at a time.)

Fast-forward a few decades, and DNA sequencing allowed the "unculturables" to step out of the shadows. Clear links emerge between microbiome patterns and obesity, diabetes, autoimmunity—even mood. Metchnikoff's hunch got biochemical legs. Finally, in 2004, a mucus-dwelling specialist appeared in a Dutch lab: *Akkermansia muciniphila*. It thrives at the interface with the gut lining, recycles mucus, fortifies the barrier, and shapes inflammation and metabolism. If Metchnikoff had met Akker, he would have grinned: Nurture the right microbe, nudge longevity.

Why did it take so long to discover friendly gut bacteria such as Akker? Before the early 2000s, studying your gut microbes was like judging ocean life by what washed up on the beach—ignoring the vast hidden ecosystems thriving below the surface. Scientists mainly relied on growing bacteria in petri dishes and broth, which meant anaerobic bacteria largely skipped the party. These oxygen-shy bacteria make up the vast majority of your gut's population, yet they were essentially invisible in early lab studies. So for decades, our picture of the gut microbiome was biased toward the small fraction of hardy microbes that didn't mind a little air.

Anatomy of the Oxygen Gradient: Why Your Colon Is a No-Oxygen Zone

As mentioned in an earlier chapter, your gut isn't uniformly oxygen-free; it has an oxygen gradient—a gradual change from some oxygen to virtually none as you move along the intestines. Picture walking from a bright, open field (your small intestine)

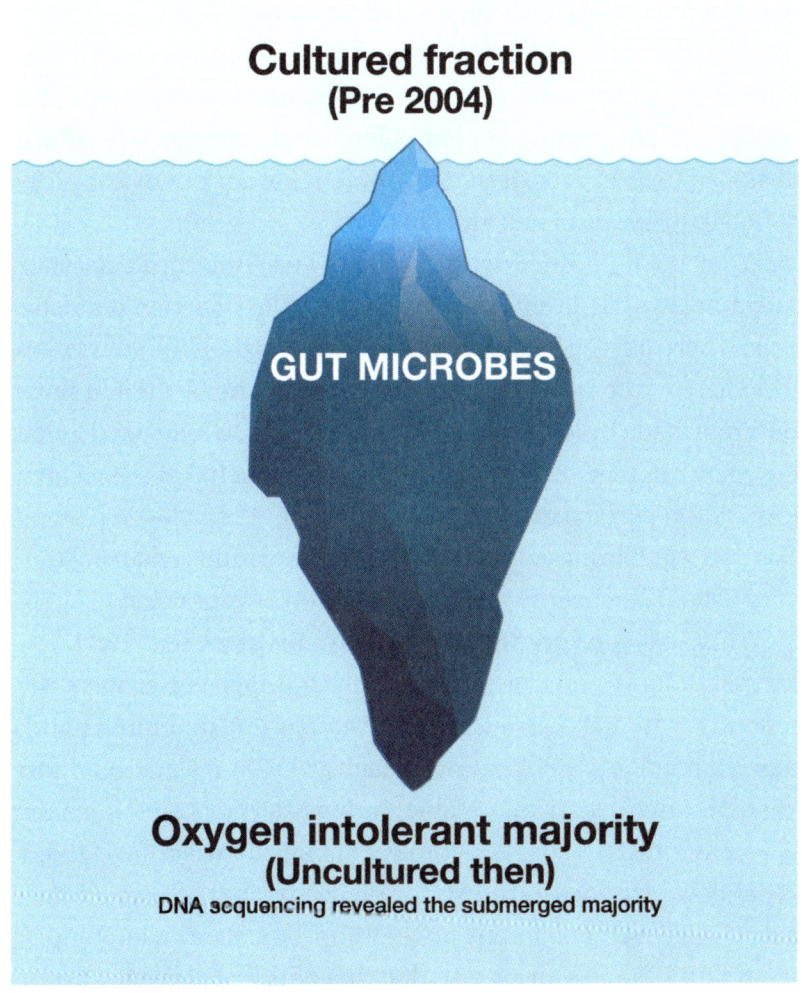

Figure 33. Iceberg blind spot in gut microbiome research. Before 2004, only the cultured fraction was visible, while DNA sequencing later revealed the vast anaerobic majority.

into a dim forest (your ileum) and then into a pitch-black cave (your colon). By the time food reaches your colon, nearly all the oxygen has been siphoned away.

The tail end of your small intestine contains a small amount of oxygen. Some of it comes from the blood vessels in the gut wall and intestinal lining, and some from swallowed air. The microbial population shifts toward the small bowel. Now, pass through the ileocecal valve—the one-way path into your large intestine—and it's as if someone shut off the oxygen supply. The cecum—the beginning of your colon—and your colon itself are designed to be oxygen-free. Any oxygen that sneaks in is rapidly gobbled up by your cells and bacteria.

Your colon is lined with a mucus layer that protects your intestinal wall. This mucus is not just a physical barrier; it's also a zone where oxygen gets consumed. The cells that line your colon (colonocytes) consume oxygen delivered by the blood and burn butyrate made by low-oxygen bacteria. In fact, when they're well fed, they ramp up oxygen consumption so much that the oxygen level at the surface drops to basically zero. It's a clever system: Your own gut lining cells act like oxygen vacuums, ensuring that very little O_2 seeps into the inner sanctum of your colon.

This oxygen gradient naturally divides the territory: Oxygen-tolerant microbes linger in the upper gut or near the mucosa, while the strictly oxygen-intolerant microbes dominate your colon's inner cavity. If each group stays in its comfort zone, this arrangement is stable. As long as your body keeps the gradient intact, the oxygen-intolerant bugs flourish—and that's great news for you. In return for their cozy, oxygen-free home, these microbes churn out a wealth of beneficial compounds, from vitamins to Gut Gems, that strengthen your gut barrier and influence your health.

The oxygen gradient doesn't just shape where microbes can live; it dictates how they make a living. Most of these anaerobic bacteria survive by fermenting whatever scraps of fiber or nutrients drift their way. But one curious resident took a different path. Instead of waiting for leftovers, it moved right into the mucus layer itself, paradoxically thriving in the very barrier meant to keep microbes at bay. That oddball turned out to be Akker, whose metabolic tricks would soon catch scientists' attention.

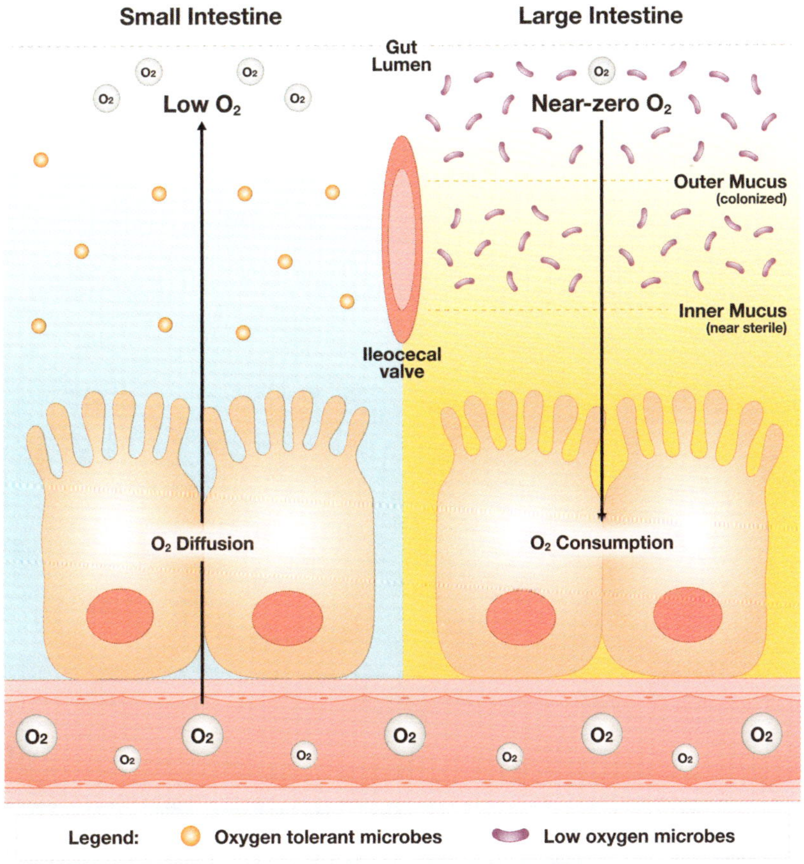

The Origin Story of Akker

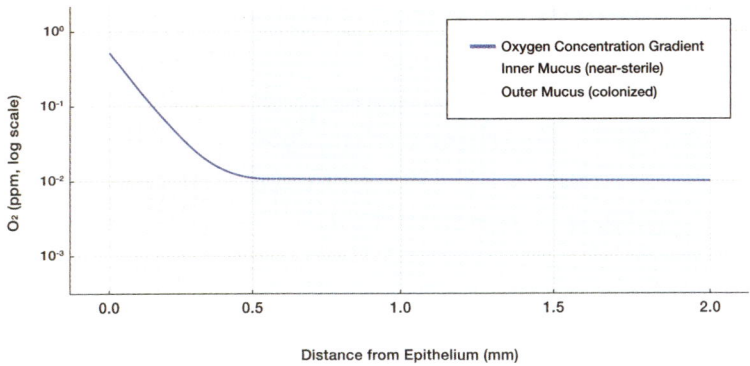

Figure 34. Diagram of the ileum and colon showing oxygen diffusion and consumption that create a sterile inner mucus layer and colonized outer mucus layer. The inset graph illustrates the steep oxygen drop within 2 mm of the epithelium.

What They Found: A Mucin Muncher with Metabolic Quirks

What makes Akker so unusual is that it can use mucin—the main protein component of mucus—as its sole source of carbon and nitrogen. Think of mucin as a gel-like matrix of sugars and protein that coats your gut lining, protecting your intestinal cells. Akker specializes in eating up this gel and breaking it down into smaller molecules. As Akker digests mucin, it turns mucus into by-products that become food for butyrate-producing bacteria living nearby. So Akker indirectly helps fuel your gut lining by enabling more butyrate-producing microbial teamwork.

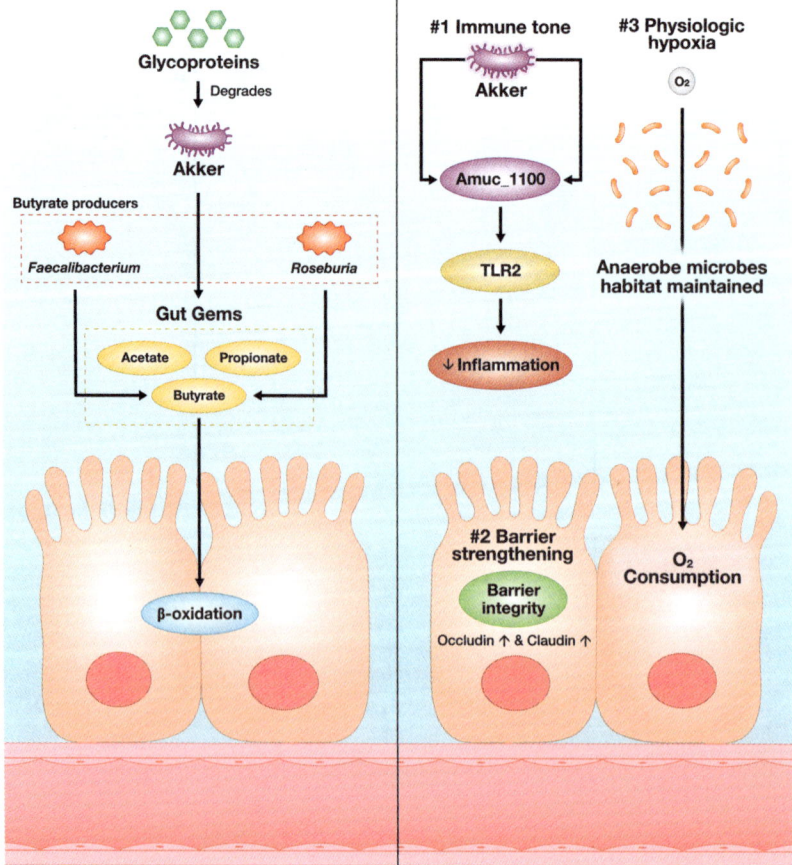

Figure 35. Mucus cross-feeding by Akker fuels butyrate producers, powering colonocytes and strengthening the barrier, immunity, and maintaining a hypoxic (low-oxygen) environment.

Why It Matters: Barrier Guardian and Metabolic Ally

Why all the fuss? As it turns out, Akker plays a pivotal role in maintaining a healthy gut environment—and, by extension, a healthy you. Scientists refer to it as a "keystone" species or even the "sentinel of the gut." Here's why: By feeding on mucin and living right on your gut lining, Akker contributes to maintaining your gut barrier on multiple fronts. This barrier isn't just physical; it's also biochemical and immunological. A strong gut barrier keeps nasty pathogens out, regulates what gets to your bloodstream, and prevents unwelcome inflammation. A sturdier barrier also supports healthier enteroendocrine signaling—including native GLP-1—which helps regulate appetite and insulin without drugs.

A well-maintained mucus layer keeps bacteria in the outer zone and prevents them from reaching and irritating the gut lining. This likely explains why Akker is linked to stronger tight junctions between intestinal epithelial cells. Tight junctions act like rivets that keep the barrier sealed. Research has shown that Akker boosts the expression of tight-junction proteins, meaning less "leakiness" or leaky gut. Next, Akker has a knack for positively influencing your immune system. Studies indicate that Akker modulates immune signaling; higher Akker abundance has been associated with increased levels of molecules that regulate inflammation. Parts of Akker, including outer membrane components, interact with receptors on our immune cells. One protein on Akker's surface, Amuc_1100, can bind to the toll-like receptor 2 (TLR2) on your gut cells, sending your immune system an "everything's fine" message instead of triggering a red alert. The result is a more tolerant immune environment with less inflammation, which is good for metabolic health.

> 📌 **Gut Concept: TLR2**
>
> - **Full name:** Toll-like receptor 2
> - **What it is:** TLR2 is a sensor protein located on the surface of many gut and immune cells. It scans for microbial signals and helps decide whether to sound the alarm or keep the peace.
> - **Why it matters:** When harmful bacteria appear, TLR2 helps trigger immune defenses. When friendly microbes such as Akker interact with TLR2 through proteins such as Amuc_1100, it sends an "everything's fine" message that keeps inflammation low while maintaining vigilance on real threats.

In the early 2010s, scientists noticed a striking pattern: lean, metabolically healthy individuals tended to have more Akker in their gut compared to those who were obese or prone to metabolic syndrome. This bug's abundance was quickly proposed as a biomarker of a "healthy gut." Multiple studies showed that giving Akker to mice that were fed a high-fat diet reduced weight gain, improved insulin sensitivity, and lowered inflammation. This single microbe led to healthier, leaner mice. Was Akker a potential silver bullet for combatting obesity and diabetes?

While these mechanisms aren't yet fully understood, a few have become clear. For one, by strengthening your gut barrier, Akker prevents the leakage of pro-inflammatory bacterial components such as LPS (lipopolysaccharide, an endotoxin) into the bloodstream. Controlling excess linoleic acid (LA) from seed oils complements this by stabilizing colonocyte membranes and the mucus layer, reducing the very leaks that drive insulin resistance. LPS in the blood is known to cause metabolic inflammation and insulin resistance. Akker helps plug the leaks, reducing the chronic inflammation that can drive weight gain and blood sugar issues.

It doesn't stop there. Akker also engages with bile acid and choline metabolism, which can influence cholesterol levels and liver health. And in an unexpected twist, Akker has been linked to better outcomes with cancer immunotherapy: Certain immune checkpoint inhibitors appear to work better when Akker is abundant in the gut—a strikingly wide-ranging impact. By modulating inflammation and metabolic hormones, this little mucus-dweller has ripple effects far beyond the colon. From barrier to brain to metabolism, the throughline is the same: Repair first; medicate less.

> 📌 **Gut Concept: Choline**
>
> - **What it is:** Choline is an essential nutrient found in foods such as eggs, liver, fish, and cruciferous vegetables. Your body uses choline to build cell membranes, make neurotransmitters such as acetylcholine (critical for memory and muscle control), and support liver function.
> - **Why it matters:** Some gut bacteria metabolize choline into compounds such as trimethylamine (TMA), which the liver converts into trimethylamine N-oxide (TMAO)—a molecule linked to cholesterol imbalance and cardiovascular risk. But not all microbes handle choline this way. Beneficial strains, including Akker, can influence choline metabolism in ways that support healthier cholesterol levels and protect the liver.
> - **Big picture:** Choline is a crossroads nutrient. Depending on which microbes process it, the outcome can be helpful or harmful. Akker helps tip the balance toward the protective side, showing how the right bacteria can turn diet into a tool for resilience rather than risk.

2008–2015: From Obscurity to the Hottest Bug in Town

For a few years after its discovery in 2004, Akker was a scientific curiosity sitting quietly in its agar tube. But by around 2008, the broader research community had begun connecting the dots—especially those studying obesity and diabetes. Large-scale DNA sequencing studies of the gut microbiome were ramping up, and one consistent finding was the inverse correlation between

Akker levels and obesity. In everyday terms, people with more Akker tended to be leaner and have better blood sugar control, while those with less Akker were often heavier or diabetic. This bug went from being unknown to a potential biomarker for metabolic health—virtually overnight.

A 2013 mouse study found that prebiotics naturally raised Akker and improved metabolism in tandem, hinting that diet can unlock the same pathway without a pill. Human cohort analyses echoed the pattern: Adults with more Akker tended to have better glycemic profiles. It was like a flurry of feel-good effects from a single intervention. Even more interesting, when the researchers fed mice a prebiotic, Akker levels rose and metabolism improved. This hinted that Akker might be a key link between diet, microbiota, and metabolic benefits.

> ### 📌 Gut Concept: Prebiotic
>
> - **What it is:** A prebiotic is a type of food your body can't digest—usually certain fibers or polyphenols—but your gut microbes can. Think of it as microbe food rather than human food.
> - **Why it matters:** Feeding the right prebiotics helps beneficial bacteria such as Akker grow stronger and multiply. For example, when researchers gave mice prebiotics, their Akker levels naturally increased, which improved their metabolism and lowered inflammation.
> - **Where to find it:** Prebiotics are abundant in onions, garlic, leeks, asparagus, green bananas, apples, and many polyphenol-rich plants.
> - **Big picture:** Prebiotics are like fertilizer for your inner garden. They don't directly nourish you, but they nourish the microbes that in turn produce Gut Gems and keep your metabolism humming.

Around the same time, human studies began reporting similar patterns. For instance, analyses of the gut microbiomes of people with type 2 diabetes or metabolic syndrome often found depleted Akker compared with healthy people. A notable 2015 study in adults with diabetes reported that those with higher Akker had lower fasting glucose and insulin than those with little or no Akker. (These associations were correlative—not causative—but the consistency was striking.) The media started picking up on the narrative that Akker was the gut bug "that keeps you thin"—oversimplified, perhaps, but grounded in emerging evidence.

By 2015, researchers were scrambling to study Akker in various disease models. Beyond obesity and diabetes, they looked at inflammatory bowel disease (IBD), autism, liver diseases, and even cancer therapies to see if Akker played a role. For example, studies in mice suggested having more Akker could reduce gut inflammation in colitis models and even slow the development of colon cancer. Meanwhile, the publication count for Akker was skyrocketing, reflecting that surge of interest.

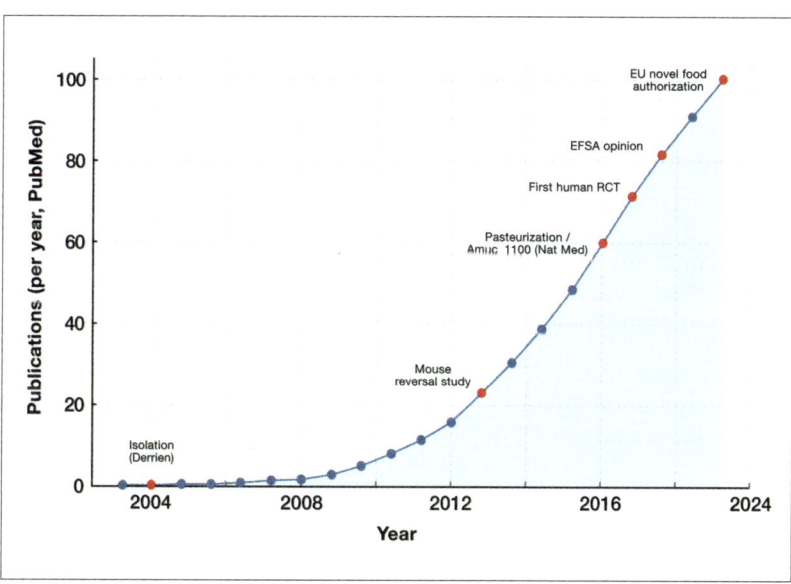

Figure 36. PubMed publications about Akker rose steeply after 2010. Milestones: 2004 isolation; 2013 mouse obesity reversal; 2017 pasteurization/Amuc_1100; 2019 first human randomized controlled trial (RCT); 2021 European Food Safety Authority (EFSA) opinion; 2022 European Union (EU) authorization.

Scientists also probed how Akker might be exerting these effects. Was it thinning the mucus, allowing beneficial immune cross talk? Were Akker's metabolic by-products influencing host metabolism? Or was Akker simply a marker of something else, like a fiber-rich diet, that was actually responsible? These were hot debate topics at conferences.

During this 2008–2015 period, another key piece fell into place: the idea that Akker might not just be a marker of health but the cause of some of these benefits. Researchers began performing fecal transplants and isolated-bacterium transfers. In germ-free mice, which have no microbes of their own, adding Akker alone could confer some metabolic benefits. That strongly suggested causality, not just correlation. If Akker was a passenger, it was one that actively grabbed the wheel and steered toward a healthier state when given the chance. The scientific community's attitude had shifted from "What's Akker?" to "How can we leverage Akker for health?"

2016–2020: From Biomarker to Probiotic Contender

If the previous years established Akker as a marker of metabolic health, 2016 onward saw the transition to "Okay, can we bottle this and use it as a therapy?" Two major breakthroughs define this period: (1) the pasteurization paradox, and (2) the first human trials.

Up until 2016, many in the scientific community assumed that if Akker were to be given as a probiotic, it would need to be delivered alive (as is generally the case for most conventional probiotics). Enter the surprise twist: Researchers discovered that pasteurized Akker was as effective as—if not more effective than—live Akker at improving metabolic health in animal models. The likely reason: Cell-surface molecules (such as Amuc_1100) do much of the signaling. That makes postbiotic formats practical and safer when the barrier is thin.

This finding was both exciting and convenient. Why convenient? Because keeping an oxygen-intolerant bug alive in a pill is challenging—imagine trying to ship a deep-sea fish in a bucket without any seawater or pressure control. But a heat-killed bacterium is shelf-stable and easier to handle. Researchers hypothesized that pasteurization might even expose or enhance certain beneficial molecules on Akker's surface, such as the protein Amuc_1100, by making them more accessible to your gut. It appears that many of Akker's benefits come from its structural components and metabolites, not from colonization and being metabolically active in huge numbers. Pasteurized Akker still carries the "goodies" that interact with your body. In microbiome lingo, this is a *postbiotic* approach—using inanimate bacterial products or cells to confer health benefits.

Buoyed by these positive animal studies, the first human trial of Akker was launched around 2016 and reported in 2019—a small but milestone randomized controlled trial that hinted at improved insulin sensitivity and liver markers. This human trial suggested Akker could indeed be a therapeutic, next-generation probiotic. It was no longer just an interesting research topic; it had real-world implications for metabolic health.

At the same time, other advances paved the way for Akker's use. One challenge was production and formulation: Akker needs oxygen-free conditions to grow, and it needs either mucin or a carefully designed medium. Researchers and biotech companies worked on refining growth media. They also explored freeze-drying and encapsulation techniques to keep Akker viable and stable for delivery. This raises the exciting possibility of making defined postbiotics: Maybe one day we can isolate the exact molecule from Akker that does the magic and use that as a drug. One study even found a specific fat from Akker that might contribute to its effects. The scientific detective work was in full swing.

By 2020, the narrative around Akker had evolved significantly. No longer just a marker of gut health, Akker was a candidate for metabolic disease therapy. Early adopters in the health community were already asking questions like, "How do I increase my Akker naturally? Should I fast? Eat certain foods? Or wait for a supplement?" Spoiler alert: You could do all the above, as we'll see next. Akker had become a probiotic celebrity, but with fame came scrutiny.

Dialing Up Your Akker—Diet and Other Levers

By now you might be wondering, "Do I have to wait for an Akker pill, or can I boost this bacterium on my own?" Great question. Research since 2016 has explored various lifestyle and dietary strategies to nudge Akker levels upward. It turns out Akker is quite responsive to diet and lifestyle changes.

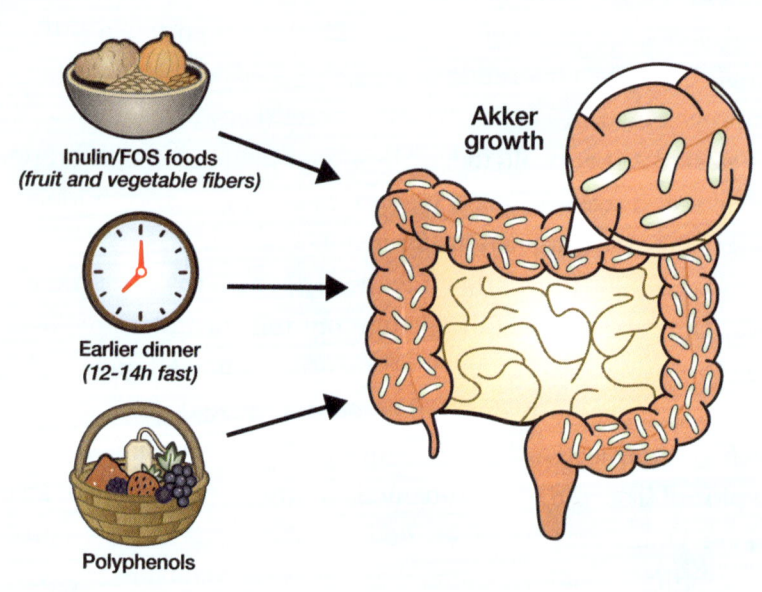

Figure 37. Dietary fiber—inulin and fructooligosaccharides (FOS)—and polyphenols feed Akkermansia; *intermittent fasting also favors its rise.*

Dietary polyphenols are antioxidant compounds in colorful fruits, tea, and wine. You probably know that red wine and cranberries are considered good for you. Part of that might be because of Akker. Because polyphenols are somewhat hard to digest, they travel to the colon and feed specific microbes. Research has demonstrated that diets rich in polyphenols (think grape skins, cranberries, and green tea) significantly promote Akker growth.

> ### 📌 Gut Concept: Polyphenols
>
> - **What they are:** Polyphenols are natural plant compounds found in colorful foods such as berries, pomegranates, tea, coffee, cacao, olives, and many herbs and spices. They're not vitamins or minerals but powerful phytonutrients.
>
> - **Why they matter in your gut:** Unlike fiber, which microbes ferment into Gut Gems such as butyrate, polyphenols act more like modulators. They're only partly absorbed in the small intestine, so plenty reach the colon, where they encourage beneficial bacteria such as Akker and suppress harmful ones. In turn, microbes break down polyphenols into smaller metabolites that calm inflammation, improve insulin sensitivity, and protect blood vessels.
>
> - **Big picture:** Think of fiber as the *fuel* and polyphenols as the *calibrators* of your gut ecosystem. Together, they power and fine-tune your microbes—one providing steady energy, the other shaping which species thrive.

For example, mice on a high-fat diet given Concord grape polyphenols had a dramatic bloom of Akker in their gut and subsequently gained less weight and had better insulin sensitivity than control mice. It appears Akker can metabolize certain polyphenol compounds or benefit from the gut environment those compounds create, perhaps by inhibiting competing microbes or by causing the host to secrete more mucus. Another strategy that's gaining attention is intermittent fasting (IF) or time-restricted eating (TRE). When you fast, even for part of the day, your gut cells produce more mucus. Akker, a mucus connoisseur, likely finds these fasting periods as buffet time. Studies have observed that during Ramadan fasting or similar regimens, Akker levels tend to increase. In mice, a daily sixteen-hour fast led to a significant rise in Akker compared with mice fed around the clock.

By adopting an eating window of eight to ten hours per day and fasting the rest, you will likely selectively boost Akker while also benefiting your metabolism directly. If your main goal is gut health and weight management, you could experiment with an earlier dinner to give your Akker a competitive edge overnight. It's far better to finish dinner earlier rather than push breakfast later, because eating at least three to four hours before bed also helps align your circadian rhythm—your body's internal clock that syncs with the day-night cycle. That way, you're not only feeding your microbes wisely but you're also training your metabolism and hormones to stay in rhythm with nature.

> 📌 **Gut Concept: TRE**
>
> - **Full name:** Time-restricted eating
> - **What it is:** TRE is a style of intermittent fasting where you eat all your meals within a limited window each day, often eight to ten hours.
> - **Why it matters for the gut:** During fasting, your gut cells shift gears. They produce more protective mucus, and oxygen levels in the colon drop, creating an ideal environment for Akker. Fasting also reduces the constant fuel supply for harmful bacteria, while helping beneficial species reset their rhythms. On top of that, fasting naturally boosts satiety hormones such as GLP-1 and PYY, giving you stronger appetite control and steadier blood sugar when you do eat.
> - **Big picture:** TRE isn't just about cutting calories—it's about creating a daily cycle of "rest and repair" for your gut and

> hormones. Think of it as giving your microbes and metabolism a cleaning shift: The gut barrier tightens, inflammation cools, and satiety hormones rise, all leaving you better prepared for your next meal.

Nuances and Caveats: Not Always a Hero?

By this point, *Akkermansia* might sound like a miracle microbe, and in many ways it is. But like any complex story, there are nuances to be aware of. Science rarely deals in absolutes, especially when it comes to something as dynamic as the gut ecosystem.

One key nuance: Context matters. In a healthy scenario, Akker's mucin-degrading activity is beneficial. However, if your gut environment is already inflamed or the mucus layer is compromised, could Akker exacerbate the problem? Some studies hint at a "double-edged sword" effect. For instance, in certain mouse studies of gut inflammation, excessive Akker was associated with worsened inflammation.

The hypothesis is that if your gut barrier is leaky or thin to begin with, too much mucin degradation could further erode the protective layer, allowing bad bugs to creep too close to the intestinal wall. This is one of the strongest arguments for starting with pasteurized Akker rather than live strains, at least until your gut barrier is repaired. Pasteurized Akker still carries surface proteins such as Amuc_1100 that calm inflammation and strengthen the mucus layer, but without the risk of excessive mucin thinning. Fortunately the concern about live Akker overdoing it seems to show up only in extreme lab conditions—such as genetically engineered mice lacking mucus genes or germ-free mice colonized with Akker alone.

There's also the issue of long-term stability. If you stop taking Akker supplements or abandon your fiber-rich diet, will your Akker population diminish? Many probiotics only transiently impact the gut unless you keep feeding them. Early signs suggest that unless you maintain the dietary habits that favor Akker, its levels could fall off after interventions stop, especially if they were low to begin with. One more nuance: interactions with other microbes. Akker doesn't live in a vacuum. Its effects can depend on who its neighbors are. If you have plenty of butyrate-producing, oxygen-intolerant microbes in the gut (such as *Faecalibacterium* and *Roseburia*), Akker's outputs will be converted to butyrate—a net win for you. But if those partners are absent (say, after antibiotics or in certain dysbiosis states), Akker might not confer the same benefit because the nutritional chain is broken.

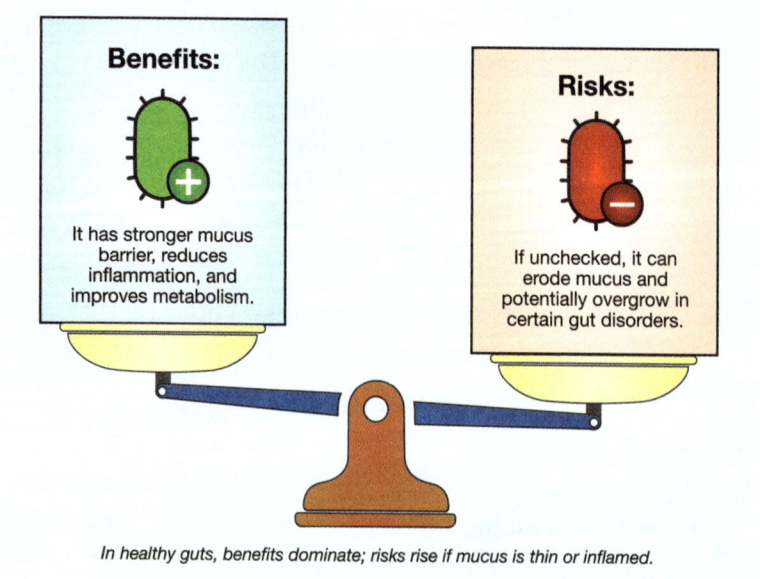

In healthy guts, benefits dominate; risks rise if mucus is thin or inflamed.

Figure 38. Akkermansia mainly supports gut health, though risks emerge when the barrier is thin or inflamed.

2021–2024: Akker Hits the Big Time

In the past few years, researchers have advanced our understanding of how Akker's mechanisms work. For example, a 2022 study reported that Akker produces tiny membrane vesicles that carry signaling molecules to the host and that a certain enzyme it makes is key to releasing a beneficial mucin fragment that communicates with our immune system. There's been exciting work on Akker's interactions with the endocannabinoid system, showing it tempers inflammation, especially in the gastrointestinal tract. A study in 2021 suggested it might alleviate features of anxiety in mice by affecting gut serotonin levels, and a 2022 trial suggested that Akker supplementation improved muscle strength in older adults. These findings paint Akker not as a one-trick pony but as a versatile organism influencing multiple body systems.

By now, public awareness of Akker has also grown. It's mentioned in health blogs, and savvy doctors or nutritionists might test for it in stool analyses as part of a personalized nutrition plan. You might see articles titled "Meet *Akkermansia*: Your Gut's Best Friend for Metabolic Health"—which, as you now know, isn't just hype.

The road ahead involves some important next steps: large-scale clinical trials for obesity, diabetes, inflammatory bowel disease, or cancer support to conclusively prove benefits in humans and get Akker from novel to recognition as a medical probiotic. Researchers are also exploring optimized combinations: Perhaps Akker works even better when paired with another beneficial microbe. Gut-based tag teams can be powerful.

It's pretty amazing to think that a microbe nobody even knew existed twenty years ago is now a front-runner in the microbiome therapeutics race. This period, 2021–2024, solidified Akker's status as a fascinating component of a healthy gut and a tangible tool we can use to improve health. The "little mucus eater that could" is now driving big changes in how we approach metabolic disease and beyond.

Gut Conquests: Your Victory Checkpoint

Today's 3-point scorecard:

1. **Move.** Walk daily (7,000–10,000 steps, or 45–60 minutes). This improves insulin sensitivity and GLP-1 signaling, amplifying Akker's effects.

2. **Feed your gut guardian.** Add a daily serving of polyphenol-rich foods (such as berries or green tea) and cut industrial seed oils high in linoleic acid (soy, corn, safflower, sunflower). Choose animal fats such as butter and ghee to nourish Akker and strengthen your gut barrier.

3. **Practice mucus-friendly fasting.** Try a gentle twelve-to-fourteen-hour overnight fast (finish dinner a bit earlier) and include a thirty-to-forty-five-minute walk to give Akker time to thrive on your gut's natural mucin supply.

CHAPTER 4
Colonocytes, Gut Gems, and Your Gut Barrier

Picture your colon cells (colonocytes) as a pack of marathoners and butyrate as their go-to fuel. Colonocytes prefer butyrate over glucose and burn about 95 percent of it locally. They pull it in through transporters and use it to make cellular energy. Why does this oxygen consumption matter? By burning butyrate so efficiently, colonocytes create a low-oxygen microenvironment at the gut surface, encouraging the proliferation of beneficial bacteria such as Akker.

> 📌 **Gut Concept: Butyrate**
>
> - **What it is:** Butyrate is a primary Gut Gem produced when friendly bacteria ferment fibers such as resistant starch, inulin, and pectin.
> - **Why it matters:** Butyrate is the preferred fuel for colonocytes, the cells that line your colon. By feeding these cells, butyrate strengthens the gut barrier, lowers oxygen levels in the colon (helping oxygen-intolerant microbes such as Akker), calms inflammation, and even influences brain function.
> - **Big picture:** Butyrate nudges L cells to release gut hormones such as GLP-1 and PYY, your body's built-in appetite killers.

Besides being a fuel, butyrate moonlights as a communication molecule. A small portion that doesn't get burned for energy heads to the cell nucleus, where it acts as a histone deacetylase (HDAC) inhibitor that blocks the activity of certain enzymes. When HDAC is inhibited, genes that promote a healthy barrier and dampen inflammation get a volume boost. This is basically butyrate telling your gut lining to reinforce itself, leading to more tight junction proteins and anti-inflammatory signals. The result is an intestinal lining that's energized, well-fortified, and inflammation resistant.

> 📌 **Gut Concept: HDAC**
>
> - **Full name:** Histone deacetylase
> - **What it is:** HDAC is a family of enzymes that tighten DNA packaging (by removing acetyl groups from histones), generally inhibiting gene activity.
> - **Why it matters in the gut:** Overactive HDAC activity can mute genes that maintain the gut barrier and temper inflammation.
> - **Butyrate's role:** Butyrate is an HDAC inhibitor—it keeps histones acetylated, DNA more open, and protective genes (tight junction proteins, barrier maintenance, anti-inflammatory signals) more active.
> - **Big picture:** Think of HDAC as a volume-down knob on gut-protective genes. Butyrate gently turns that knob up again, helping your lining stay sealed, calm, and resilient.

The end result of this butyrate-powered system is a harmonious gut ecosystem. Your colonocytes stay hyped up on their preferred fuel, using oxygen so fast that the environment stays comfortably oxygen-free for your fiber-fermenting bacteria. Those bacteria, in turn, continue producing butyrate and other Gut Gems that benefit your body, creating a positive feedback loop, as illustrated on the following page.

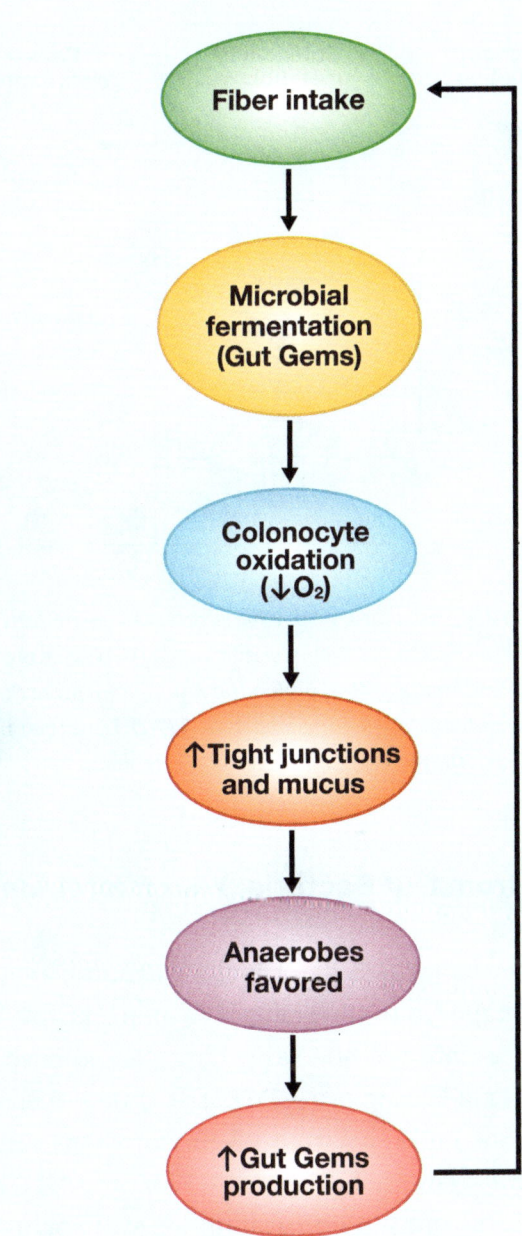

Figure 39. The repair loop: Fiber fuels microbes to produce Gut Gems; colonocytes burn those Gut Gems, oxygen levels drop, the barrier tightens, and anaerobes thrive.

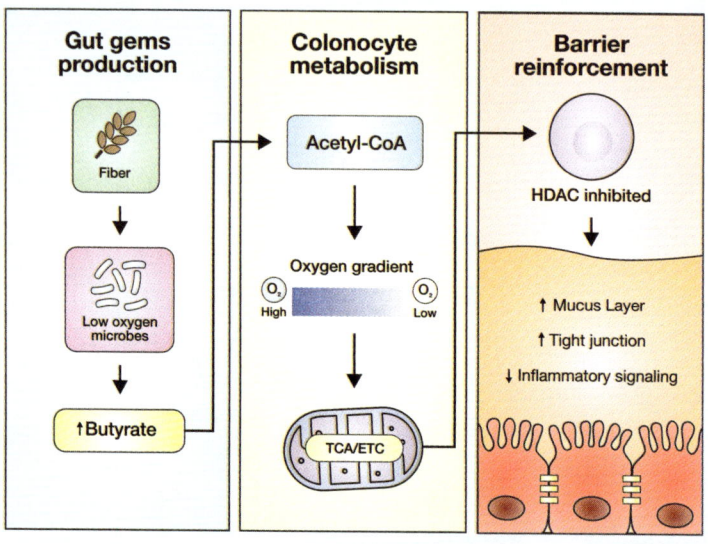

Figure 40. Butyrate from dietary fiber fuels colonocytes by converting into acetyl-CoA, which enters the tricarboxylic acid (TCA) cycle—also called the citric acid or Krebs cycle—within the mitochondria. In this cycle, acetyl-CoA is oxidized, producing NADH and FADH$_2$, carrier molecules that shuttle high-energy electrons.

Gut Gems from Gut Bacteria: Your Microbiome's Love Letters

Your Gut Gem molecules don't just sit around; they actively signal and shape your physiology. Acetate, propionate, and butyrate can all bind to special sensors on your cells called G-protein–coupled receptors (GPCRs)—think of these as doorbells on various cells that ring when Gut Gems press them. Different GPCRs (such as GPR41, GPR43, and GPR109A) are found on cells in your gut lining, immune system, and even on hormone-producing cells.

How it works: When Gut Gems ring these doorbells, they trigger changes in the host cell. In the colon and lower small intestine, Gut Gems stimulate enteroendocrine cells (hormone-releasing cells sprinkled in your gut lining) to secrete hormones such as GLP-1 and PYY. GLP-1 and PYY help regulate gut motility and send "I'm full" signals to your brain. So, yes, the fiber your microbiome ferments into Gut Gems can indirectly influence your appetite and digestion speed!

> 📌 **Gut Concept: GPCRs**
>
> - **Full name:** G-protein–coupled receptors (GPCRs)
> - **What they are:** GPCRs are cell-surface "switchboards" that turn outside chemical signals into inside actions.
> - **Where they are:** They are found on gut L cells, immune cells, colonocytes, adipose tissue, and some neurons.
> - **Why they matter:** Gut Gems activate specific GPCRs leading to GLP-1 and PYY release, tighter junctions in the gut lining, and a lower inflammatory tone.

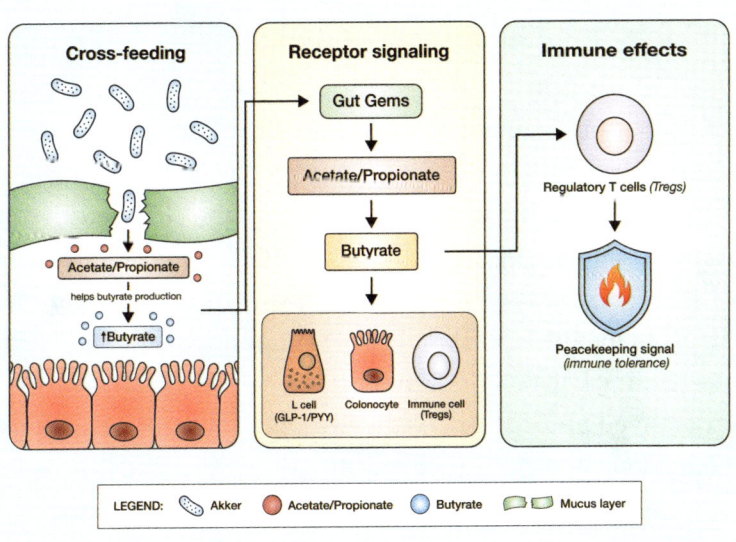

Figure 41. Butyrate and propionate promote regulatory T cells while dampening pro-inflammatory activity, fostering immune tolerance.

Gut Gems	Main cell types	Key outcomes		
		GLP-1/PYY	Barrier tightening	Tregs/ immune tone
Acetate[1]	L cells, immune cells, colonocytes	✔ Increase in GLP/PPY	✔ Increase in tight junctions and mucin	✔ Tregs increase; immune tone is calmer
Propionate[2]	L cells, immune cells, colonocytes	✔ Increase in GLP/PPY	✔ Increase in tight junctions and mucin	✔ Tregs increase
Butyrate	Colonocytes, immune cells, some L cells	✔ Increase in GLP/PPY	✔ Strong through HCAR2 and HDAC	✔ Tregs increase; anti-inflammatory signals increase

[1] Acetate circulates systemically; cross-feeds butyrate producers
[2] Propionate is heavily taken up by the liver; it also cross-feeds butyrate producers

Figure 42. Matrix showing how acetate, propionate, and butyrate act on gut and immune cells to trigger hormone release, strengthen the barrier, and promote immune tolerance

Another important function of Gut Gems is directed at your immune system. They encourage the production of regulatory T cells (Tregs), which are peacekeeper immune cells that reduce inflammation. At the same time, Gut Gems can dampen the activity of inflammatory cells, meaning fewer hair-trigger reactions. That means less friendly fire at your gut barrier and fewer leaks feeding back into inflammation.

Balanced pools of Gut Gems are key. You want a Goldilocks scenario: not too little, not too much. Each Gut Gem plays a unique role. Acetate can travel in the bloodstream and even reach the liver, where it may influence cholesterol metabolism and gluconeogenesis, the process of converting glucose into glycogen for energy storage. Propionate is known to be taken up by the liver and has effects on glucose production. Butyrate mostly stays in the colon, fueling colonocytes and reinforcing the local barrier. Together, this trio of Gut Gems ensures multiple benefits: energy for your colon lining; gut-brain signals for appetite and motility; and immune modulation for a tolerant, non-inflamed gut environment.

📌 Gut Concept: Tregs

- **Full name:** Regulatory T cells
- **What they are:** Tregs are a specialized type of immune cell whose job is to keep the immune system from overreacting.
- **Why they matter:** Tregs are boosted by Gut Gems such as butyrate and propionate. They tell the immune system to tolerate friendly microbes and lessen inflammation. Without enough Tregs, the gut can slip into autoimmune or inflammatory overdrive.

Your colonocytes are glued together by tight junctions. These junctions determine what passes through the gaps—mostly nothing larger than a water molecule. If they're nice and snug, you have a well-regulated gut filter. If they loosen up ... well, that's when you get into "leaky gut" territory (more on that soon).

📌 Gut Concept: Leaky Gut

- **What it is:** Leaky gut is a condition where the junctions between cells in your intestinal lining loosen too much, allowing substances that should stay inside the gut (like food particles, bacterial fragments, and toxins such as LPS/endotoxin) to slip into the bloodstream.
- **Why it matters:** When these "foreign" molecules leak out, the immune system reacts as if under attack. This sparks chronic low-grade inflammation that can ripple through the whole body, affecting metabolism, mood, and even brain function.

- **Drivers:** Drivers include diets high in LA-rich seed oils, which make cell membranes fragile and prone to oxidation, and low fiber intake, which limits Gut Gem production. The result is higher oxygen levels in the colon, and fewer friendly microbes.
- **Fix:** The fix is more fermentable fiber, reduced LA consumption, and simple movement to tighten the seals.

Above this cellular seal is the mucus layer, a two-tiered gel-like blanket made by goblet cells, which are specialized cells in your gut lining. The mucus has a dense inner layer attached to the epithelium, thick enough that bacteria can't easily penetrate it. As a result, it stays relatively bacteria-free, providing a protective coating over your intestinal cells. The outer mucus layer, in contrast, is more porous. It's the zone where friendly bacteria mingle—with our friend Akker being a prime example. They generally don't reach the epithelial cells because of the inner layer's firm barrier.

Now, where do Gut Gems come into play here? They can act on goblet cells through those GPCR "doorbells" or by inducing signaling molecules such as prostaglandins, to ramp up the secretion of mucin. Gut Gems also strengthen your chemical barrier by enhancing production of antimicrobial peptides (AMPs). AMPs are tiny proteins, such as defensins and cathelicidins, that function as natural antibiotics.

📌 Gut Concept: AMPs

- **Full name:** Antimicrobial peptides
- **What they are:** They are small protein "bullets" made by your gut lining and immune cells to keep microbes in check. They don't wipe out all bacteria but selectively target the troublemakers (opportunists and pathogens) while sparing friendly species.

- **Why they matter:** AMPs act as part of your gut's built-in defense system. When your barrier is healthy, AMPs are released in just the right amounts to stop bad bugs from overgrowing. But if your gut lining is damaged or inflamed, AMP production can be disrupted, tilting the balance toward dysbiosis.
- **Big picture:** Think of AMPs as your gut's neighborhood watch—always patrolling, keeping order, and making sure the friendly bacteria can thrive without being crowded out by opportunists.

Butyrate, for example, can nudge intestinal cells to crank out more AMPs, helping keep the microbial community in check by making sure no one species, especially a pathogenic one, overgrows. Meanwhile, secretory immunoglobulin A (sigA) is an antibody that your gut immune cells secrete into the mucus. Its job is to bind to microbes and prevent them from sticking too closely to your gut wall or from invading.

📌 Gut Concept: Secretory Immunoglobulin A

- **Full name:** Secretory immunoglobulin A (sigA)
- **What it is:** SigA is an antibody made by your gut's immune cells and secreted directly into the mucus layer that coats your intestines.
- **Why it matters:** SigA acts like a front-line security team. It binds to microbes and food particles, preventing them from sticking too closely to your gut wall or breaking through the barrier. Instead of killing microbes outright, sigA tags and blocks them, keeping the peace without sparking full-blown inflammation.
- **Gut Gem connection:** Gut Gems such as butyrate can boost sigA release, strengthening this protective shield.

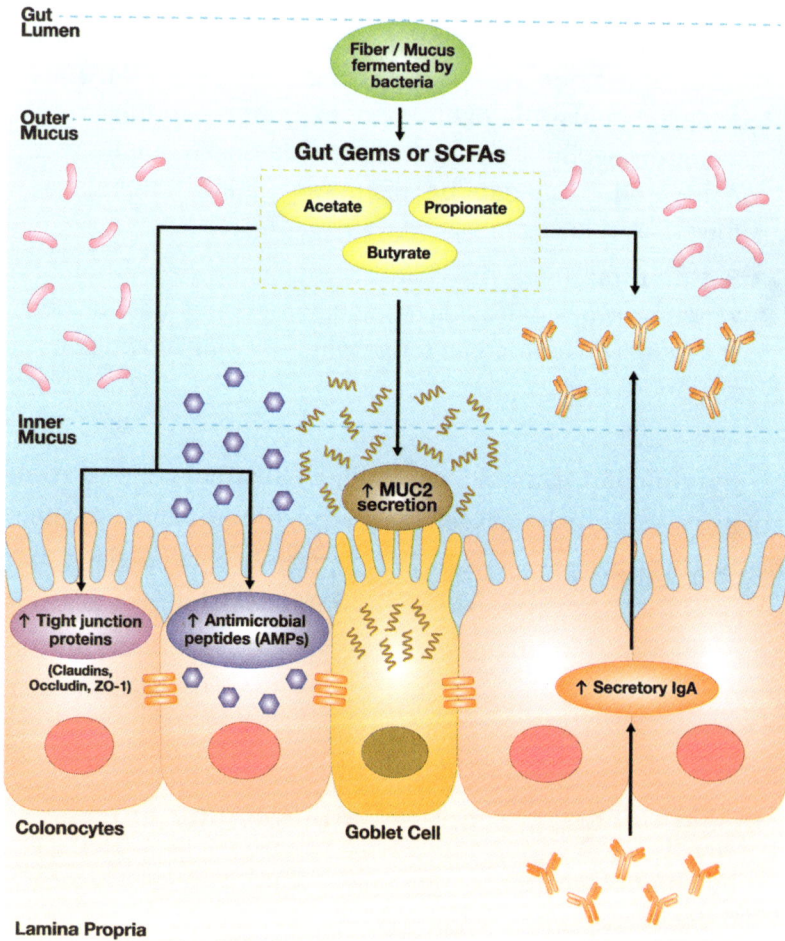

Figure 43. Dietary fiber and mucus fermented by gut bacteria produce the Gut Gems acetate, propionate, and butyrate. These metabolites fuel colonocytes, which support the production of antimicrobial peptides and reinforce tight junction proteins that seal gaps between cells. Butyrate also stimulates goblet cells to increase MUC2 secretion, thickening the mucus layer that shields the intestinal lining.

How Colonocytes Keep It Oxygen-Free: The Hypoxia Heroes

Ever wonder how your gut stays mostly oxygen-free when technically it's inside a well-oxygenated body? It's not magic—it's metabolism. Your colonocytes are hypoxia heroes, constantly maintaining an oxygen gradient that keeps the intestinal environment ideal for friendly bacteria. We touched on this earlier; now let's dive a bit deeper into that mechanism and why it's so crucial.

When colonocytes consume butyrate, they create a phenomenon called "physiological hypoxia" in the gut lining. *Mechanism recap:* By burning butyrate in your mitochondria, colonocytes use up oxygen and effectively scavenge oxygen from inside your large intestine.

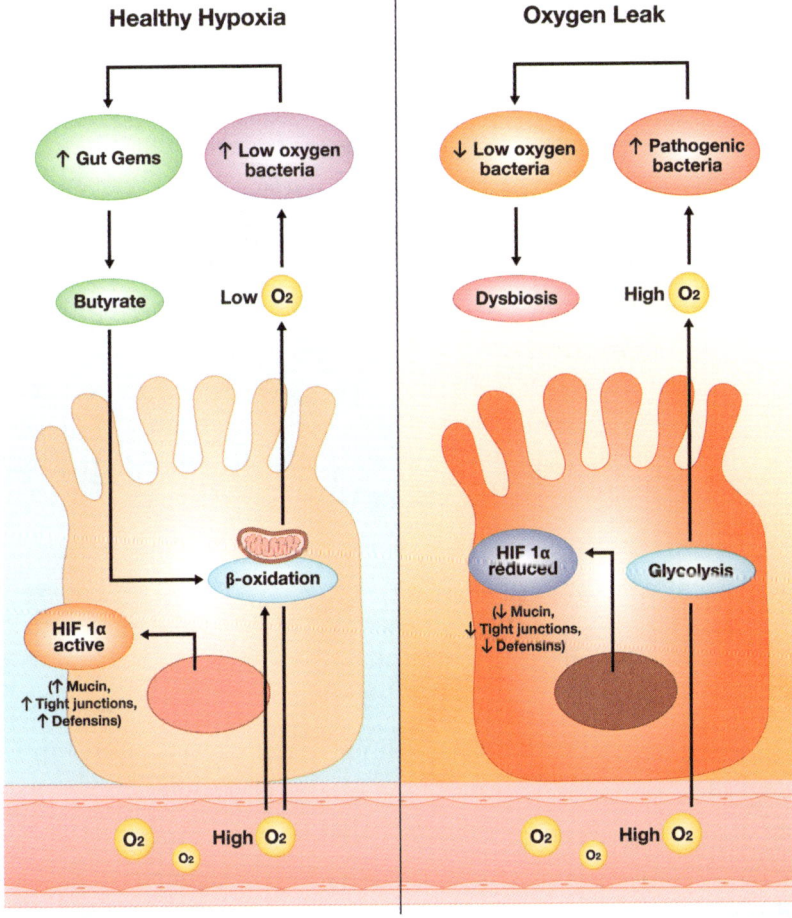

Figure 44. Colonocytes maintain a low-oxygen environment via butyrate metabolism; glucose use reduces oxygen consumption, favoring pathogens.

This reduces the oxygen concentration in the immediate area to trace levels—perfect for oxygen-intolerant microbes. Your body essentially creates an oxygen tension divide at the colon mucosal interface. The gradient is steep: just a tiny bit deeper into the mucus or inside the colon and oxygen levels drop to near zero. Meanwhile, on the other side of the colonocytes, in the underlying blood vessels, oxygen is plentiful.

One major benefit of this low-oxygen zone is the activation of a protein called hypoxia-inducible factor 1-alpha (HIF-1α). HIF-1α is like a master switch that flips on when oxygen is low.

> 📌 **Gut Concept: HIF-1α**
>
> - **Full name:** Hypoxia-inducible factor 1-alpha
> - **What it is:** It's a protein inside your cells that acts like a low-oxygen sensor. Under normal oxygen levels, it's constantly broken down. But when oxygen drops—as it naturally does in the colon—HIF-1α stabilizes and switches on.
> - **Why it matters in the gut:** Once active, HIF-1α switches on genes that help your gut lining adapt to low oxygen and stay strong. These include genes for mucin production (thicker mucus), tight junction proteins (tighter seals between cells), and defensins (a type of AMP).
> - **Big picture:** HIF-1α is like your gut lining's emergency preparedness coach. It senses when oxygen is low and rallies defenses to reinforce the barrier, keeping pathogens out and your friendly microbes safe.

Under normal oxygen conditions, HIF-1α gets constantly degraded (imagine a timer that resets whenever there's too much oxygen). But when oxygen levels drop—as they do thanks to butyrate metabolism—HIF-1α stabilizes and accumulates in the cell's nucleus.

What does HIF-1α do? It switches on a suite of genes that help the gut adapt to low oxygen and strengthen barrier defenses. For instance, HIF-1α target genes include those that increase mucin production, tight junction proteins, and defensins (a type of AMP), all contributing to a tougher barrier. It even nudges cells to rely more on glycolysis, a way of generating energy without needing oxygen.

By maintaining this low-oxygen environment, colonocytes also handicap potential bad microbes. Many dangerous pathogens are oxygen-tolerant microbes. This means they can survive without oxygen—but boy do they love it when oxygen is around, as in a high-oxygen, inflamed gut. However, in a healthy, low-oxygen colon environment, these pathogens lose their edge. They're forced to compete on the same playing field as the slow-and-steady fermenters, which they're not good at. Essentially low oxygen keeps the playing field level, so beneficial anaerobes remain dominant.

What Can Go Wrong: Leaky Gut and Inflammation on the Warpath

Leaky gut is the popular term for increased intestinal permeability, meaning the junctions between cells aren't as tight as they should be. This allows microbes and their toxic tidbits, such as LPS, to get into areas where they don't belong—such as your bloodstream or deeper tissues. Your immune system, ever the vigilant guard, immediately senses danger and can go into overdrive. The result? Inflammation, inflammation, inflammation. This inflammation can be localized, causing gut symptoms, and/or systemic triggering issues elsewhere.

As noted earlier, leaky gut occurs when the intestinal lining becomes overly permeable, allowing bacteria and toxins to leak through. This sparks chronic inflammation that can ripple through the body.

A mild leaky gut may be the link between poor diet, microbiome changes, and diseases such as obesity, type 2 diabetes, or even neurological conditions. Similar to a low-level infection,

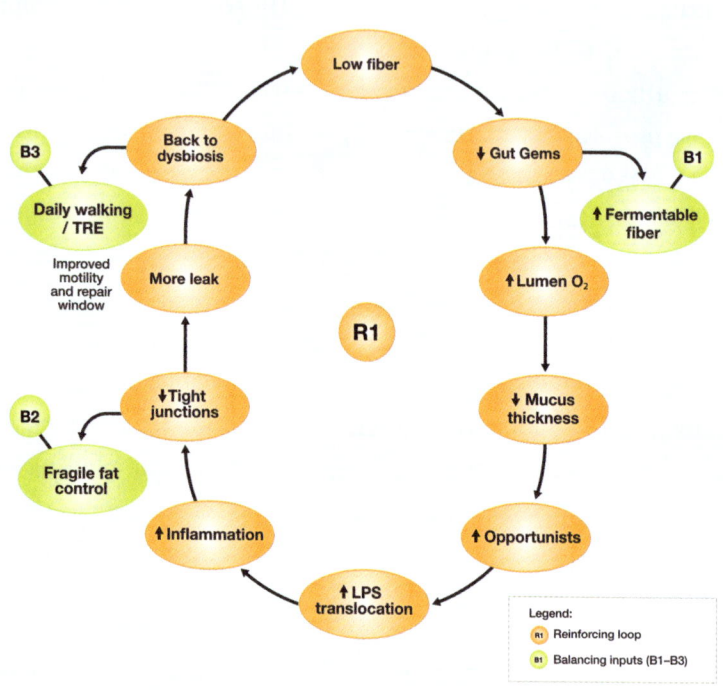

Figure 45. Low fiber intake drives a reinforcing loop of dysbiosis and leakiness, while high fiber, low LA intake, walking, and TRE act as balancing inputs that break the cycle.

your immune system is never fully at peace because microbial molecules are regularly penetrating the gut wall. This chronic immune activation can alter how you metabolize food and how your hormones function. It can stress toxin-filtering organs such as the liver, which becomes overburdened, contributing to conditions like fatty liver disease. Not to mention, chronic inflammation is a known risk factor for cancer. A leaky, inflamed colon environment could, over years, increase the risk of colon polyps or cancerous changes because of constant cell regeneration.

In everyday terms, if you've been dealing with issues such as bloating, food sensitivities, or brain fog, focus on barrier support. This could be as simple as eating groats for breakfast, adding fermented food or resistant starch, and staying hydrated. As a bonus, you might be surprised to see improvements in seemingly unrelated areas—clearer skin, better mood, fewer aches. That's the beauty of gut health: Fix the foundation and the whole house is stronger.

Your Gut Health Checkpoint

You've made it through the nitty-gritty of colonocytes, Gut Gems, and the gut barrier—give yourself a high five! Now let's turn knowledge into action.

Consider this your personal checkpoint on the path to stronger health. Below is today's 3-point scorecard—three actionable takeaways from this chapter. Complete each mini-goal to claim a win for your health:

1. **Ditch the seed oils.** Do a quick scan of your kitchen and plate. Most packaged snacks, salad dressings, and restaurant fryers are laced with seed oils high in LA, such as soy, corn, sunflower, and safflower. These fragile fats oxidize easily and weaken gut cell membranes, feeding inflammation. Swap them for stable fats such as butter, ghee, tallow, or coconut oil, and sub in whole foods instead of packagod ones.

2. **Tighten your eating window.** Try compressing your daily eating into an eight-to-ten-hour block—a simple form of TRE. By giving your gut a long nightly rest, you lower inflammatory load, improve microbial rhythms, and allow colonocytes to repair junctions without constant food stress. Start by pushing breakfast a little later or dinner a little earlier, and let water, black coffee, or tea carry you through the fasting hours.

3. **Walk it in.** Try to get in thirty to sixty minutes of walking each day. Walking after meals helps shuttle glucose into

muscles, keeps insulin sensitivity high, and pushes more fermentation substrate to your colon microbes. Walking also increases blood flow to the gut lining, supports motility, and reduces stress hormones that otherwise chip away at barrier integrity. It's low tech, low cost, and one of the most reliable methods for gut repair.

Remember, while GLP-1 drugs such as semaglutide mute your appetite, they do nothing to rebuild your gut barrier. They act as a Band-Aid rather than a baseline fix. By repairing the circuit instead—through controlling fragile fats consumption, simple movement, and added fiber—you can increase your tolerance with no bloating, gas, or distension.

CHAPTER 5
The Seed-Oil Catastrophe: How Seed Oils Changed Your Gut's Ecosystem

Over the past century, industrial seed oils—cheap fats pressed from soybeans, corn, and other crops—have taken over our diets. These oils are loaded with linoleic acid (LA), a polyunsaturated omega-6 fat. Back in chapter 1, we gave PUFS like LA a new name, "fragile fats," because of how unstable and easily damaged they are. We'll use that term a lot in this chapter since they are at the center of the story. Thanks to mass production and aggressive marketing, we now consume thousands of times more fragile fats than our great-grandparents did.

This chapter makes a bold claim: The rapid rise of LA-rich seed oils has reshaped your colon's ecology, disrupting the harmony between your gut cells and their microbial roommates, including Akker. We'll connect the dots from seed oils to colon biology to microbial misbehavior—and ultimately to what it all means for your waistline, liver, and beyond. By the end of this chapter you'll see how something as mundane as cooking oil can derail metabolism, why avoiding these fats (and restoring Akker) changes the game, and what to do next.

Most of us grew up hearing that vegetable oils were "heart-healthy" replacements for butter and lard. So how could these oils possibly be a health catastrophe? Context is key. The turn of the twentieth century saw an explosion in processed foods and modern manufacturing. In 1911, the multinational consumer goods company Procter & Gamble introduced Crisco, a hydrogenated cottonseed-oil product that was the first major industrial seed oil sold as food. Soon cheap soybean, corn, sunflower, and safflower oils flooded the market. Fast-forward to today and you'll find seed oils in everything from salad dressings to fast-food fries. In fact, by some estimates, these oils contribute up to a fifth of all calories in the modern American diet—a colossal shift from a hundred years ago. Our gut and metabolism have been enrolled in a giant, unplanned dietary experiment— one that our mucus layer, Akker, and colonocytes never voted for.

Here's the crux: Your body was never meant to handle such an onslaught of unstable polyunsaturated fats at the levels we now consume—especially not when these fats are chemically enhanced and hidden in thousands of ultra-processed foods. We're going to explore how this new-normal level of fragile fat intake might be quietly sabotaging your colonocytes and tipping your microbiome into disarray. It's a tale of chemistry gone rogue—but it's not all doom. Understanding the problem is the first step to fixing it. By the end of this chapter you'll have learned some simple tweaks to put things right. (Don't worry— we're not expecting you to churn butter or hunt whales for fat.)

A Century of Seed Oils: From Crisco to Corn Chips

It all started with a problem: too much cotton, not enough butter. In the late 1800s, there was an excess of cottonseed, an industrial waste product. Solution? Turn it into food. By 1911, Crisco (hydrogenated cottonseed oil) hit American kitchens, marketed as a pure, modern alternative to lard and butter. Housewives were told this snow-white shortening would make for flakier pies and healthier families. And it sold like hotcakes. Soon after, soybean oil came along. By the 1940s and '50s, soybean oil was king, surpassing butter, lard, and even cottonseed. The food industry loved these oils: They were cheap, plentiful, and—thanks to hydrogenation—could be molded into margarines and shortenings that mimicked butter. Convenience and profit drove a dietary revolution.

World events gave seed oils another boost. During wartime and the postwar boom, animal fats were rationed and expensive, so people turned even more to plant-based substitutes. Then came the great saturated fat panic of the 1960s and '70s. The physiologist Ancel Keys and other experts of the day pushed the "heart-healthy" message: Cut back on animal fats to fight heart disease. The answer on grocery shelves? Bottles of "pure vegetable oil"—soybean, corn, safflower—flaunting their cholesterol-free virtues.

Food manufacturers reformulated products, and fast-food chains famously switched from beef tallow to vegetable oil for frying. Unfortunately, partially hydrogenating those oils created harmful trans fats that quietly pervaded our food until bans came decades later. But even as trans fats disappear from ingredient lists, the core issue remains: Our diets are drowning in liquid polyunsaturated fat, especially LA.

To grasp the magnitude of change, consider this jaw-dropping stat: Per capita soybean oil consumption in the United States skyrocketed more than a thousandfold from 1909 to 1999. In 1900, the average American ate virtually no industrial seed oil; today, these fragile fats make up an estimated 7 to 8 percent of our daily calories.

The following graph shows how US oil intake shoots up like a rocket in the mid-twentieth century. Meanwhile, rates of obesity and metabolic diseases began creeping up in parallel. Of course, seed oils were not the only culprit here; many other factors came into play—high-fructose corn syrup, ultra-processed foods, synthetic food additives, portion sizes, and increasingly sedentary lifestyles. But the timing of the seed-oil surge and our health decline is suspiciously aligned. By 2020, US obesity prevalence had swollen to over 40 percent of adults, up from about 13 percent in 1960.

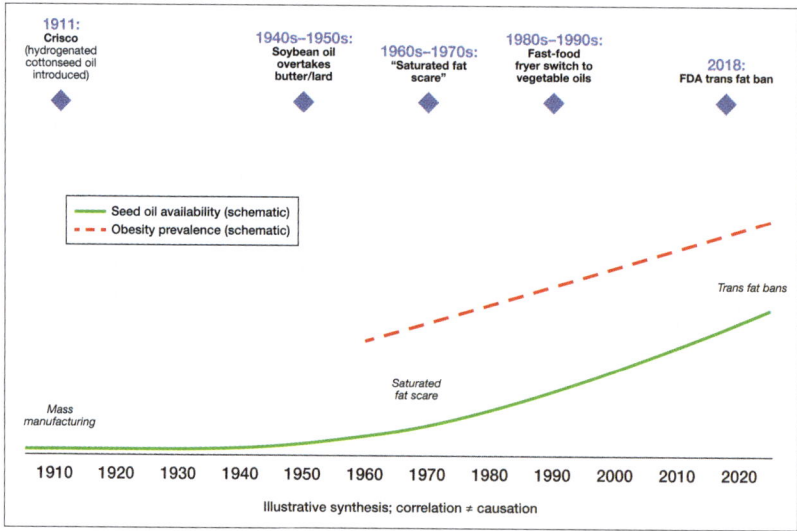

Figure 46. Timeline of US seed-oil adoption (1911–2020) showing key product milestones, rising oil availability (green line), and parallel obesity prevalence (red line)

In short, we changed the fuel mixture for our body's engine without full knowledge of the long-term consequences. The rest of this chapter explores one crucial consequence: what all that LA-rich oil may be doing to your colon. Why the colon? Because that's where trillions of microbes live and where dietary fats (and their nasty breakdown products) can directly influence your health. It turns out the colon is like the canary in the coal mine for dietary change. So, let's put on our miner's helmet and shine a light on the chemistry happening in those crispy fried foods and salad dressings.

Unstable Fats Equal Toxic Soup: Chemistry 101

Seed oils come from nature, but by the time they reach your plate, they've often been refined, bleached, heated, and exposed to air—a perfect recipe for oxidation. That process generates a burst of free radicals and peroxides. Fragile fats have two double bonds in their structure, making them highly prone to peroxidation (the scientific term for reacting with oxygen). When you heat these oils to frying temperatures, they start breaking down within minutes. Researchers found that when vegetable oil is heated to about 365°F for just a half hour, it forms large amounts of 4-hydroxy-2-nonenal (4-HNE). If that chemical name sounds ominous, it should—4-HNE is basically a toxic aldehyde, a reactive compound that can wreak havoc in your body.

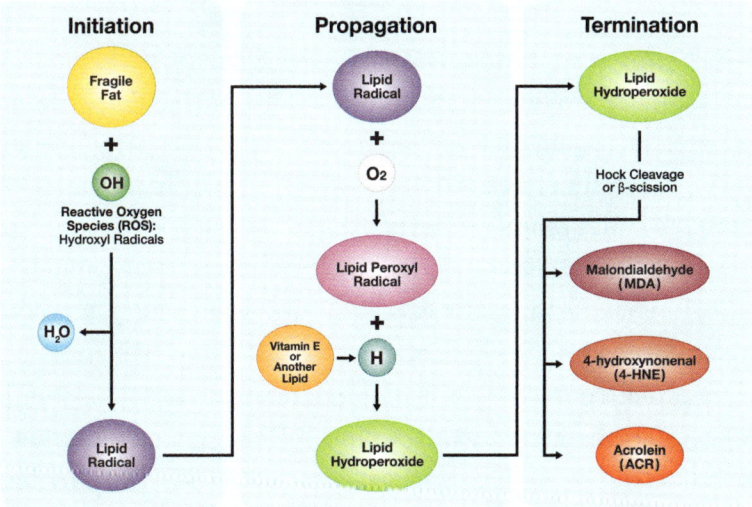

Figure 47. Lipid peroxidation pathway from fragile fats, showing initiation, propagation, and termination into toxic aldehydes

📌 Gut Concept: 4-HNE

- **Full name:** 4-hydroxy-2-nonenal (4-HNE)
- **What it is:** It's a toxic aldehyde formed when seed oils rich in fragile fats such as LA are heated to cooking temperatures, especially over 365°F.

> - **Why it matters:** 4-HNE is highly reactive. Once formed, it can bind to proteins, DNA, and cell membranes, disrupting normal function. In the gut, it damages colonocytes, weakens your gut barrier, and fuels inflammation. Systemically, 4-HNE has been linked to oxidative stress, mitochondrial dysfunction, and chronic diseases such as atherosclerosis and neurodegeneration.
> - **Big picture** This is one of the clearest reasons why fragile fats (see Gut Concept: LA) are so dangerous. When they break down, they don't just fail to protect you—they actively generate a toxic by-product in the form of 4-HNE.

Let's break that down in everyday terms. Overheated oils cause lipid peroxides to form—unstable molecules that can decompose into smaller nasties such as aldehydes. Among them, 4-HNE is the superstar villain. It's been called "highly toxic" by scientists and is readily absorbed when you eat fried foods. What does it do? 4-HNE loves to react with proteins, DNA, and other critical molecules in your cells. Picture a molecular wrecking ball smashing into the delicate machinery of your cells.

Another troublemaker is malondialdehyde (MDA), a smaller aldehyde formed from oxidized fats, often used as a marker of rancidity and oxidative stress. These aldehydes not only form in the oil—they soak into the food being fried. Here's a kicker: These toxic compounds accumulate with each cycle—think of a restaurant deep fryer in which oil is used repeatedly all day. And unlike some toxins that get detoxified in the liver, aldehydes such as 4-HNE hit your gut lining before your body has a chance to neutralize them. They can also slip into circulation, contributing to systemic inflammation. In short, an LA-rich oil under heat is a factory for oxidative toxins.

Ultra-processed foods often contain oils that were heated during manufacturing to extrude that chip, puff, or cereal—creating pre-oxidized oils. Even storage can cause some oxidation

The Seed-Oil Catastrophe: How Seed Oils Changed Your Gut's Ecosystem

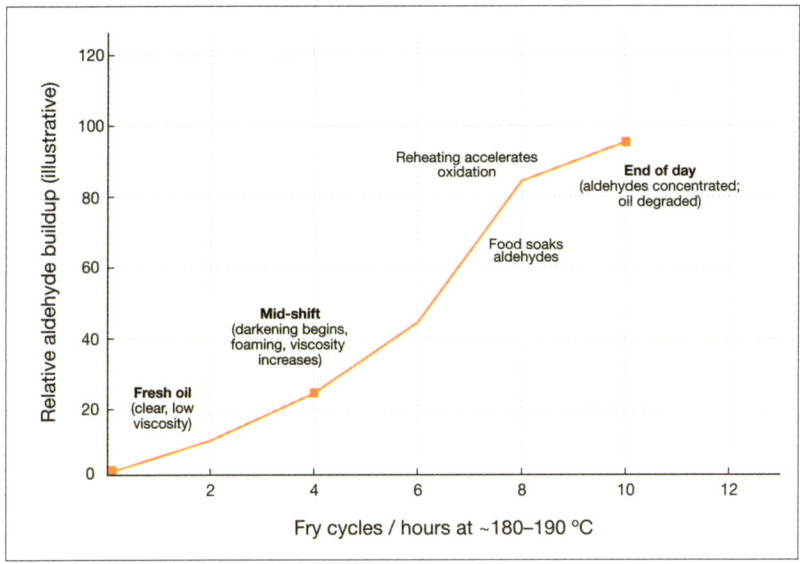

Figure 48. Illustrative chart showing aldehyde buildup across repeated frying cycles, with notes on oil oxidation, darkening, reheating effects, food soaking aldehydes, and end-of-day degradation

if the oil isn't handled carefully. All these factors mean your gut environment is facing oxidative stressors it rarely encountered in the preindustrial diet. Traditional fats such as butter, ghee, tallow, and coconut oil are mostly saturated or monounsaturated; they're more stable under heat, producing far fewer nasty by-products. But with high fragile fat oils, we've changed the game.

So, to sum up, fragile fats are double-bond rich oils that, when exposed to heat and oxygen, turn into a toxic soup of peroxides—4-HNE, MDA, and others. If you're thinking, "This doesn't sound good," you're right. But knowledge is power. Now you know that not all oils are benign, especially once the flames are crackling.

How Seed Oils Hurt Gut Cells

Your colonocytes normally live in symbiosis with your gut microbes, forming a barrier and gobbling up nutrients such as butyrate. But when oxidized seed oils enter the scene, it's like tossing a grenade into an orderly barracks. As mentioned, one of the chief offenders is 4-HNE, which damages colonocytes by disrupting mitochondria—the tiny energy-producing factories inside cells that burn fuel. As a result, colonocytes lose their ability to generate energy efficiently. 4-HNE can attach to and disable key enzymes in this process, effectively sapping the colonocyte's ability to burn butyrate. This leads to a cascade of trouble: When colon cells can't burn butyrate well, they start struggling to meet their energy needs and may resort to less efficient pathways.

One observable consequence is that colonocytes reduce the expression of the transporter that brings butyrate from the gut's inner space, or lumen, into the cells. Imagine a factory that stops importing raw materials because it can't process them efficiently anymore. Why does this matter? Butyrate isn't just any fuel—it's the fuel for healthy colon cells, and burning it has special benefits. Perhaps the most immediate hit from 4-HNE and similar lipid peroxides is on the tight junctions between your colonocytes. Experiments show that 4-HNE suppresses the expression of tight-junction proteins, resulting in barrier disruption. As discussed in the previous chapter, simply introducing 4-HNE in mice was shown to weaken gut-barrier proteins and allow bacterial components such as LPS to leak into the bloodstream, sparking inflammation.

So, now we have a trifecta of colonocyte injury: mitochondrial dysfunction (less energy, less butyrate use), barrier disruption (loose tight junctions, leaky gut), and endoplasmic reticulum (ER) stress—the cell's version of a distress signal. There's one more piece to the puzzle: oxygen. What happens when 4-HNE and oxidative stress derail butyrate metabolism? The colonocytes consume less oxygen; local oxygen levels creep up; and HIF-1α, sensing more oxygen, becomes destabilized.

Without HIF-1α, your colonocytes produce fewer of the protective factors that help maintain the mucus layer and barrier function. In essence, your gut lining loses its oxygen shield.

Research confirms this mechanism in high-fat diet models: Impaired mitochondrial fat burning in colon cells leads to higher epithelial oxygen levels and loss of that hypoxic barrier. It's a bit like your gut's eco-friendly, low-oxygen zone turning into a rusty, poorly sealed oxygen-rich zone. And guess who loves that extra oxygen? The wrong kind of gut bugs.

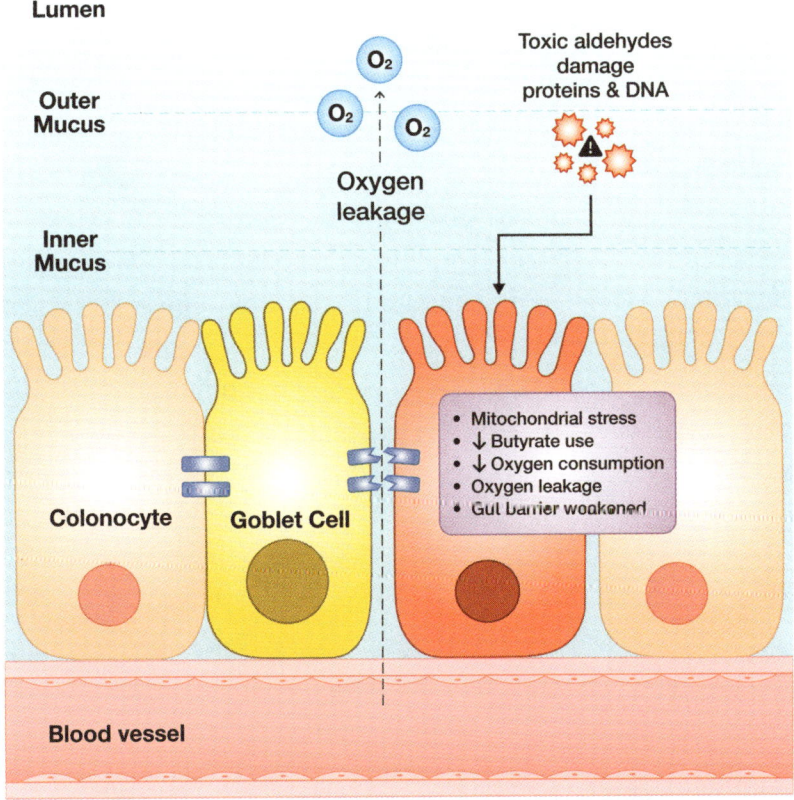

Figure 49. Cutaway of the colon lining showing how toxic aldehydes injure colonocytes, including mitochondrial stress, reduced butyrate use, oxygen leakage, and weakened gut barrier

Microbes Gone Mad: Dysbiosis from Oxidative Stress

As we know, your gut microbiome thrives under low-oxygen conditions. Most of your beneficial gut bacteria flourish in the cozy, oxygen-free depths of your intestines. But when seed oils tilt your colon's environment, the microbial balance shifts. Elevated oxygen levels in the colon lumen act like a welcome mat for a different group of microbes: facultative anaerobes, which are bacteria that can use oxygen when it's around. This group includes many members of the Proteobacteria phylum—think E. coli and its cousins. Under normal conditions, these guys are kept in check. But with elevated levels of oxygen and some extra nutrients, they're ready to go.

Indeed, studies have found that when colonocyte metabolism is impaired, it can lead to an expansion of Proteobacteria in the gut. It's worth noting that dysbiosis linked to diets high in fragile fats or oxidized fats may contribute to systemic issues far removed from your gut. A leaky gut can drive insulin resistance, liver fat accumulation, and even affect our mood and immune responses. Some researchers suspect that the modern epidemic of metabolic conditions might involve this gut microbial shift—essentially, our Western diet fertilizes a pro-inflammatory microbiome that then makes us prone to obesity and diabetes. Seed oils could be a significant piece of that puzzle, working in tandem with excess sugars and low fiber to create a perfect storm.

Bottom line: Your gut's ecosystem thrives on the fuel and environment you give it. Flood it with unstable fats and oxygen, and you select for a very different crew of microbes than if you feed it fiber and keep it anaerobic. Next, we'll zoom out and see how these gut-level changes might connect to the bigger picture of disease trends and, crucially, how to balance this teeter-totter back in the right direction.

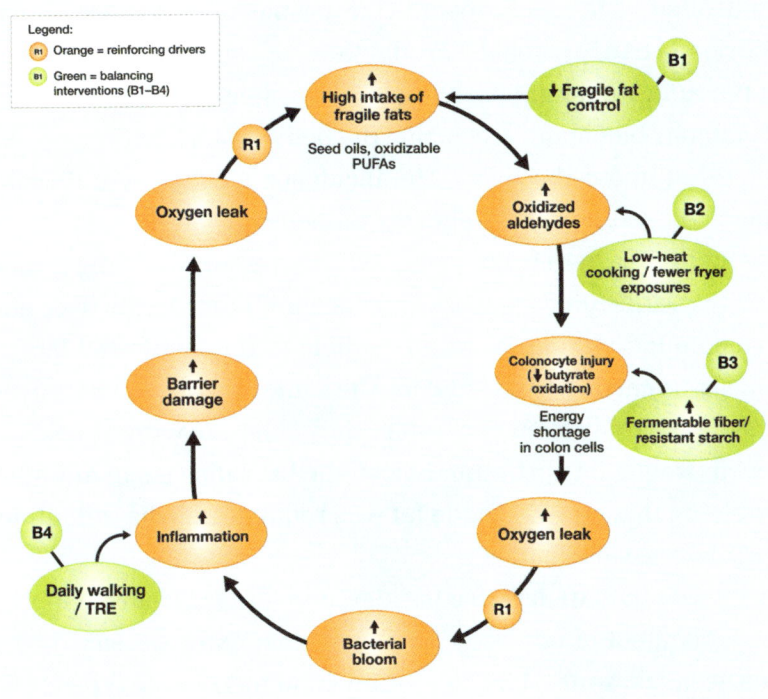

Figure 50. Fragile fat-derived aldehydes trigger a reinforcing loop of colonocyte injury, oxygen leakage, inflammation, and Proteobacteria bloom.

Big Picture: Obesity, Liver Trouble, and the Seed-Oil Debate

Although the evidence linking them is still evolving, the rise of seed oils correlates strikingly with the rise of obesity and metabolic diseases in the twentieth century. As mentioned, Americans in 1900 ate virtually no industrial seed oils; today these oils are ubiquitous. Researchers have reported a strong correlation between LA intake and obesity prevalence in the United States.

In mouse experiments, diets high in soybean oil (which is about 50 percent LA) led to more weight gain and fat accumulation than diets high in saturated fat, even when calories were controlled. The mechanism? One proposal is that fragile-fat overload can increase production of endocannabinoids—compounds that ramp up hunger and fat storage. Too much fragile fat may biochemically prime the body to store fat.

What about the liver? The incidence of fatty liver disease has exploded alongside obesity. Some researchers point a finger at diets high in fragile fats. In rodent models, adding fragile fats to the diet tends to worsen fat accumulation in the liver and promote inflammation, whereas diets rich in saturated fats or omega-3s cause less liver fat for the same calories. There's even older research (from the 1980s and '90s) showing that diets low in fragile fats prevented alcoholic liver disease in animals, implying that excess fragile fat was required for the inflammatory damage to occur.

While human data are trickier, one thing is clear: The fragile fat content of our body fat has dramatically increased over the decades. Your fat tissue composition reflects the types of fat you eat, and modern Americans have about triple the fragile fat in their bodies compared with people in the 1960s. This could influence how our fat cells function and how much inflammation they produce, since oxidized fragile fat in adipose tissue can attract immune cells. In short, our bodies are literally built differently at the molecular level than those of our ancestors.

To be clear, excess calories from any source will cause weight gain. Seed oils often come packaged in calorie-dense junk foods, so is it the oil that's at fault or the doughnut as a whole? Most likely both. Sugar and refined carbs also surged in the twentieth century. And many ultra-processed foods are a witch's brew of high LA, high-fructose corn syrup (HFCS), and low fiber, making it hard to pin blame on one ingredient alone. So, when we talk about seed oils correlating with obesity or fatty liver, remember it's part of a broader dietary pattern. Seed oils may aggravate metabolic issues, especially in the context of a Western diet, but they're rarely acting alone.

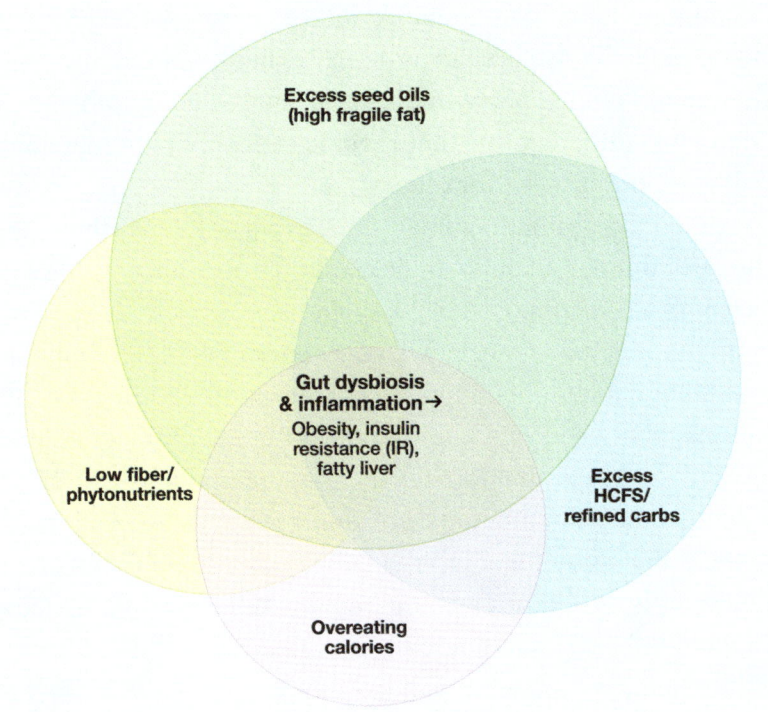

Figure 51. Overlapping Western diet risks converge on gut dysbiosis, fueling obesity, insulin resistance, and fatty liver.

Another confounder is that health-conscious people often avoid saturated fats, choosing more seed oils instead, but they also tend to practice other healthy habits. In studies, this can make high seed-oil use look beneficial when the real driver of better outcomes may be factors such as eating more vegetables or replacing something clearly worse, such as trans fats. This is why epidemiological studies can be paradoxical. That said, emerging human studies are intriguing. Some controlled trials suggest that lowering seed-oil intake and replacing them with, say, monounsaturated fats or carbs can reduce inflammation markers and improve insulin sensitivity. There's also interest in whether diets high in seed oil drive up oxidized LDL—the "bad" cholesterol implicated in heart disease—more than other fats do, given fragile fat's susceptibility to oxidation. And recall those nasty aldehydes such as 4-HNE. They've been detected at higher levels in people with diseases such as colon cancer and ulcerative colitis, hinting that chronic exposure may contribute to disease processes over time.

To be fair, some mainstream experts argue that seed oils are fine or even beneficial for cardiovascular health, focusing on outcomes like LDL cholesterol reduction rather than the gut-level effects we've been exploring. The heart-health-versus-metabolic-health debate can be confusing. It's possible that seed oils could marginally lower heart disease risk factors while simultaneously nudging up diabetes risk. Or perhaps moderate amounts are fine but excessive use, especially when oils are heated, is a problem. Our view, based on the evidence, is that caution is warranted. Where does this leave GLP-1 drugs? While they can suppress appetite and tweak metabolism, they don't repair colonocytes, prevent leaky gut, or restore Akker. Plus, once the medication is stopped, appetite returns; the "wire" reconnects. Fix the circuit—lower LA, rebuild the mucus layer, walk daily, feed your microbiome—and satiety emerges naturally.

Taking Back Control: Practical Tips to Outsmart Seed Oils

Enough science—let's talk action. How can you enjoy your meals without marinating your colon in oxidized LA? The good news: You don't have to abandon delicious food or live off boiled broccoli. A few strategic tweaks can dramatically cut your fragile-fat intake and support your gut health:

- **Use the Mercola Health Coach app (Seed Oil Sleuth).** Download the free app and try the Seed Oil Sleuth feature. It's a high-tech way to navigate the minefield of fragile fats in your diet. The app quizzes you on your eating habits, spots seed oils in places you'd never expect, and guides you step-by-step toward safer swaps. Most people are shocked when they see just how much of these fats they're eating—and how seed oils sneak into nearly every packaged or restaurant food. The app makes it simple and personal, helping you avoid the traps that labels often conceal.

 Scan this QR code to get FREE access to the Mercola Health Coach app. This tool allows you to log your meals, track your macronutrient ratios, and monitor your progress over time.

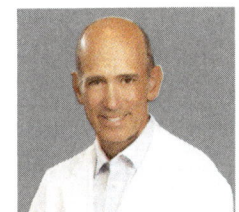

- **Choose better fats.** Ideal options include traditional fats such as butter, ghee, tallow, and coconut oil, which are rich in saturates and far less prone to oxidation when cooking. Be cautious with olive oil and avocado oil: While in their pure form they can be healthy in small amounts, studies show that up to 80 percent of bottles on the market are adulterated with cheap seed oils. If you use them, make sure you trust the source. Also avoid nut oils, which are highly unstable under heat.

- **Dodge the fryer—or fry smart.** It's no surprise: The worst seed-oil offenders are deep-fried foods from restaurants and packaged snacks. That basket of fries or potato chips has likely been fried in oil used repeatedly over multiple shifts. If your main goal is to lose weight, cutting out commercial fried foods is a quick win, eliminating a huge source of empty calories and oxidative stress. Read labels too: Many crackers, cookies, and roasted nuts are made with soybean or sunflower oil. Opt for products that use healthier oils or are oil-free.

- **Balance your fats.** Historically, humans ate omega-6 and omega-3 fats in a closer ratio—maybe 2:1 or 3:1. Today's Western diet can be 10:1 or even 20:1 in favor of omega-6. The solution isn't to chase supplements but to rebalance naturally. While omega-3s (EPA and DHA) produce fewer inflammatory by-products than omega-6s, over 90 percent of omega-3 supplements on the market are heavily processed, rendering the final product into something far from the natural oils you get from the whole fish. It's far better to get your omega-3s from fresh seafood like wild-caught Alaskan salmon, mackerel, herring, sardines, and anchovies. Natural foods provide fats in their intact form, along with antioxidants that help protect them.

- **Fiber, fiber, fiber.** We've talked so much about butyrate because it's central to colon health. When you feed your gut bugs fiber, they churn out Gut Gems that heal your gut lining, bolster mucus, and signal your immune system to chill out. A high-fiber diet effectively counterprograms many of the harmful effects of seed oils. Some fibers, such as pectin in apples or beta-glucan in oats, have even been shown to bind and expel some fat by-products. Polyphenol-rich foods (pomegranates, cranberries, green tea, cocoa) are especially friendly to Akker. And don't forget fermented foods such as yogurt, kefir, sauerkraut, and kimchi, which help introduce beneficial microbes and metabolites. Try this: Pick one simple swap—maybe trade that afternoon snack of chips for a handful of carrots or add a side salad with dinner. Consider making a daily fiber pledge. Your microbiome will respond in kind.

- **Avoid smoke points.** If you use vegetable oils, treat them gently. Never heat oils past their smoke point—that bluish smoke is a sign you're generating a swarm of peroxides. For instance, unrefined sunflower oil has a low smoke point; it's better for drizzling, not frying.

Refined oils have higher smoke points, but remember that high heat still produces aldehydes even if you don't see smoke. Low-and-slow cooking methods such as baking, steaming, and stewing use less oil and cause less oxidation than deep-frying or searing. A practical tip: Preheat the pan first, then add oil right before the food, so the oil doesn't break down as quickly. Or better yet, sauté in a splash of broth or wine and add a bit of oil for flavor at the end. These little hacks reduce the total heat exposure of oils.

- **Eat mostly single-ingredient foods.** Build meals from meat, fish, eggs, vegetables, fruit, tubers, and legumes. Fewer barcodes usually mean fewer hidden seed oils.

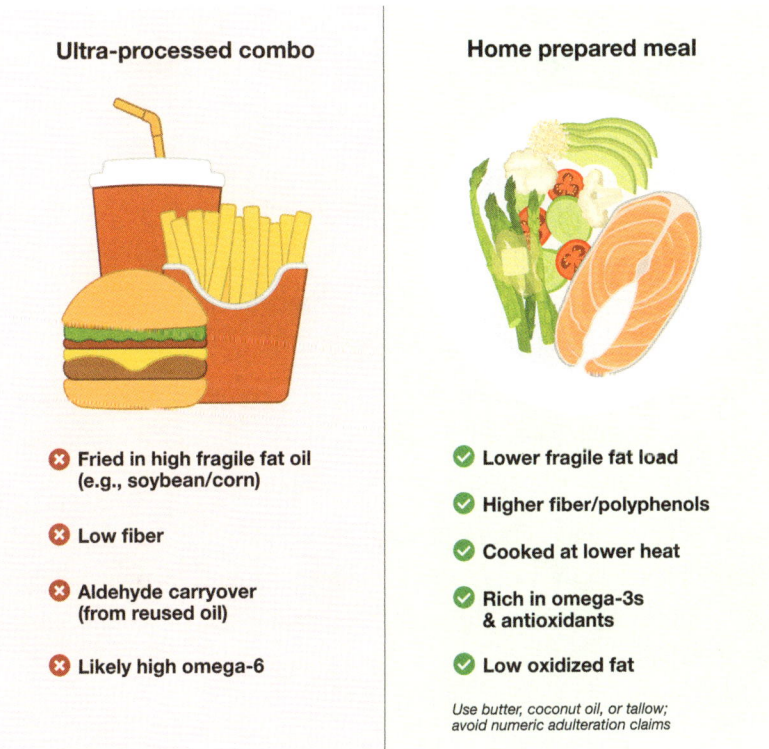

Figure 52. Fast food has more fragile fat and less fiber and antioxidants than a home-cooked meal.

So, where to begin? First, prioritize. Identify the biggest source of seed oils in your diet and tackle those first. For a lot of people, it's restaurant food (especially fast food) and packaged snacks. Start by cooking at home one day a week with healthier oils. Or if you love salads, switch to homemade dressing with olive oil. If your main goal is gut health, consider adding a daily probiotic or a prebiotic fiber supplement to amplify those Gut Gems. Before we wrap up, here's a fun challenge: Open your pantry and grab one packaged food you eat often. Fire up the Seed-Oil Sleuth in the Mercola Health Coach app and see if it can spot something better for you. Can you find a similar product with healthier oils—or even make a better version yourself? Treat it like a little project. You may just stumble onto a new favorite.

Weight-Loss Conquests: Your Victory Checkpoint

Today's 3-point scorecard (tackle these and give your colon a high five):

1. **Increase fiber.** Add one extra serving of fiber per day this week to feed beneficial gut bacteria.
2. **Add antioxidants.** Include a high-polyphenol food in at least one meal or snack per day.
3. **Go for probiotics.** Try one fermented food this week, such as sauerkraut, kefir or yogurt (ideally homemade from organic, grass-fed, raw milk), or kimchi.

The takeaway: Ozempic and other GLP-1 drugs can make you eat less, but they don't rebuild your gut wall, prevent oxygen leak, or restore Akker. Cutting fragile fats, walking, and eating real food do.

CHAPTER 6
GLP-1 and Akker's Secret Weapon

This chapter shows how L cells, Akker, and a diet low in fragile fats keeps hunger at bay—without needles. Your intestine is lined with tiny sensor cells that keep tabs on what you eat. Meet the L cells, a special-ops team of cells mostly camped out in your ileum (with a sizable squad in the colon). Their numbers increase as you move down the intestines, with a substantial proportion found in the colon, where oxygen levels are low.

Although these cells make up only a tiny fraction of the gut lining, they are mighty, each equipped with receptors that can detect nutrients from your meal. How do they "taste" anything? L cells have G-protein–coupled receptors (GPCRs)—molecular locks that only specific nutrient "keys" can open. When a glucose or fat molecule comes along and fits into one of these locks, the L cell instantly responds. L cells also play a direct role in mechanosensing in the GI tract. Research shows that L cells possess mechanosensitive ion channels that allow them to detect mechanical stimuli from the stretching, pressure, and flow caused by intestinal contents.

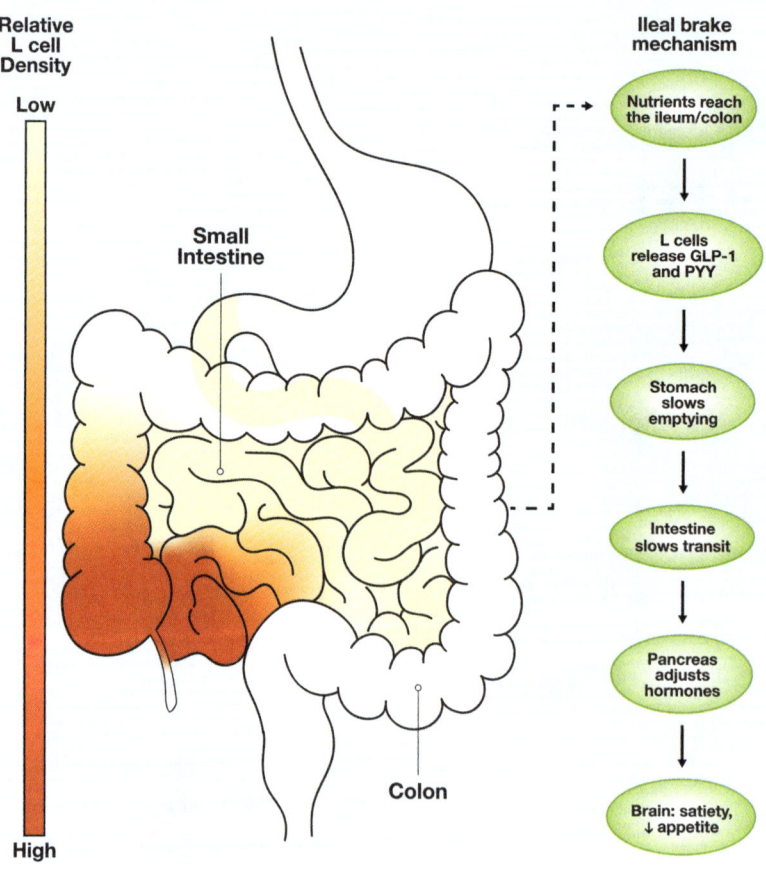

Figure 53. The ileal "brake"—L cells concentrated in the distal gut—releases GLP-1 and PYY to slow digestion and promote satiety. These cells are rare but powerful, and they are most abundant in the ileum and colon, where oxygen levels are low.

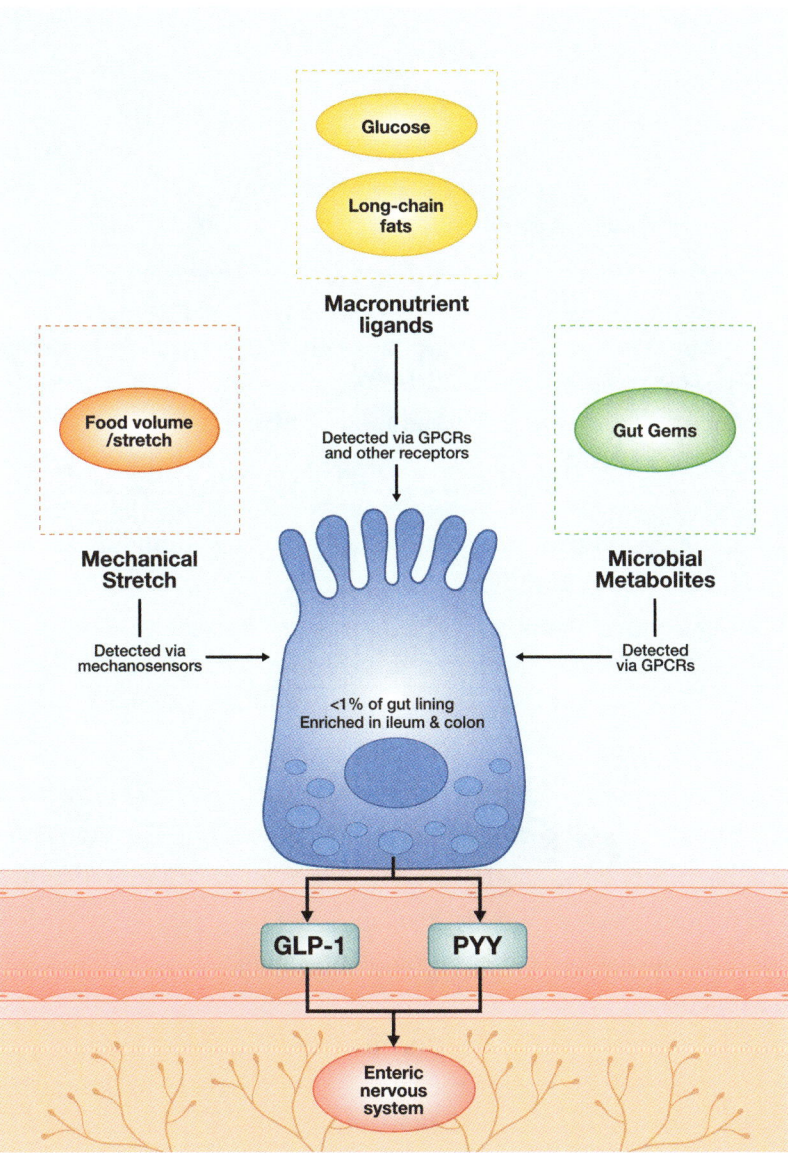

Figure 54. L cells sense nutrients such as glucose and long-chain fats, along with microbial metabolites (Gut Gems). In response, they release GLP-1 and PYY, which act on the enteric nervous system to regulate digestion and appetite.

> 📌 **Gut Concept: L Cells**
>
> - **What they are:** L cells are specialized cells scattered along your intestine, with the highest numbers in the ileum and colon. They make up less than 1 percent of your gut lining, but they pack a punch.
> - **How they work:** L cells act like microscopic "tasting booths." They carry GPCRs, which are nutrient-sensing receptors that detect glucose, fats, and even the physical stretch caused by food. When a nutrient key fits into a receptor lock, the L cell responds instantly.
> - **What they release:** Once triggered, L cells secrete powerful hormones such as GLP-1 and PYY. These satiety messengers tell your brain you're full, slow digestion, and help balance blood sugar.
> - **Big picture:** Think of L cells as your gut's special-ops signal corps. They are small in number, strategically placed, and crucial for balancing appetite and metabolism.

Once an L cell's receptors detect a nutrient, the cell releases hormonal messengers into your bloodstream, including GLP-1 and PYY. Because L cells are strategically positioned as a last checkpoint, food is mostly broken down by the time it reaches them. What's left are trickier nutrients, such as fiber and protein fragments. Your body can respond to these "late arrival" nutrients by secreting hormones that fine-tune digestion and appetite. This is sometimes called the "ileal brake," when L cells sense a heavy load and signal your stomach and intestines to slow down.

Translation: Smart Brakes, Not Sledgehammers

The slow, low-oxygen environment of the colon means bacterial fermentation by-products hang around longer, increasing their chance to interact with L cells. The colon's thick mucus lining also brings bacteria and L cells into proximity while maintaining a protective barrier.

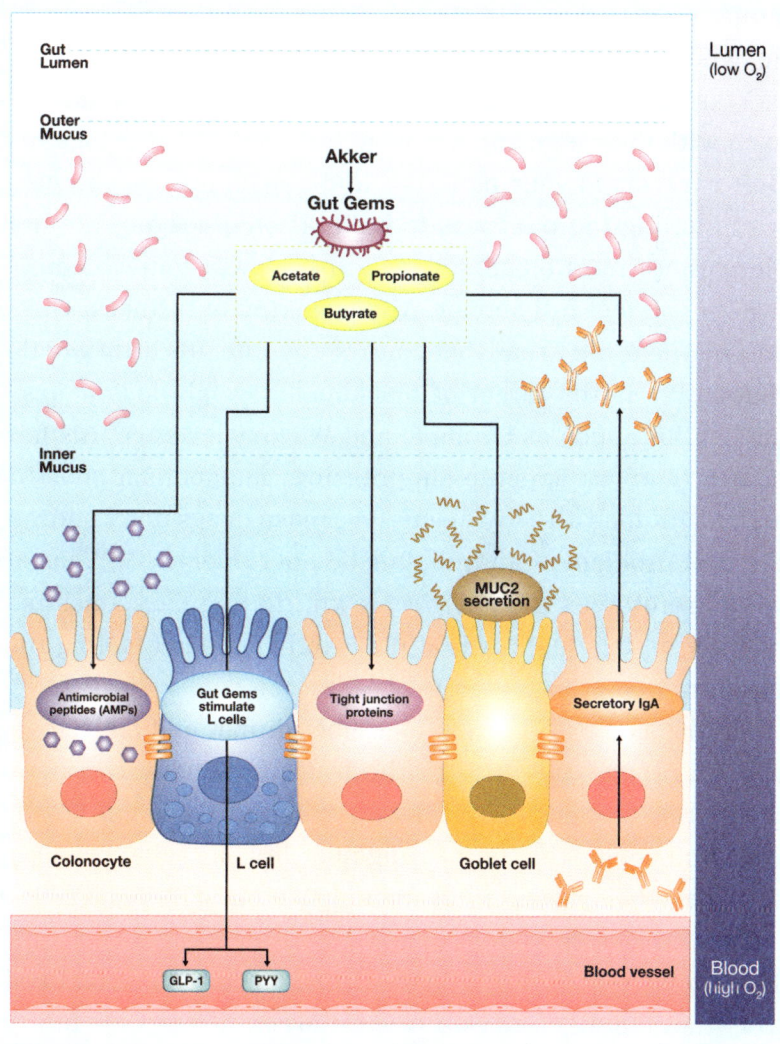

Figure 55. Colon cutaway showing the two-layer mucus with Akker-producing Gut Gems (acetate, propionate, butyrate) that diffuse to L cells, stimulating GLP-1 and PYY release. Antimicrobial peptides, tight junction proteins, secretory IgA, and MUC2 (a major mucous protein) secretion together maintain barrier defense.

GLP-1 and PYY: Your Dynamic Duo for Appetite and Sugar Control

So, what do these gut hormones do once released? GLP-1 and PYY are like the Batman and Robin of appetite regulation—each with their own superpowers but even stronger together. GLP-1 travels to your pancreas and boosts insulin secretion while telling the pancreas to hold off on glucagon, the hormone that raises blood sugar. It also slows stomach emptying, so you feel full sooner. And speaking of fullness, GLP-1 acts on the brain areas that control appetite. It's little wonder that GLP-1 is the target of blockbuster weight-loss drugs—medications such as Ozempic and Wegovy leverage this hormone's natural appetite-suppressing, metabolism-boosting actions. But, as already discussed, these drugs don't address the root problem of an unbalanced microbiome. PYY, meanwhile, reinforces the gut slowdown, dialing back intestinal motility and giving you that pleasantly satisfied feeling that discourages second helpings.

Ever had a protein-rich, high-fiber dinner and noticed you weren't rummaging through the fridge later? You can thank the extra PYY and GLP-1 released from all those gut L cells. Research shows that fermenting fiber in your colon produces Gut Gems that trigger L cells to pump out more PYY and GLP-1, leading to reduced appetite and less weight gain over time. That's a big reason why high-fiber diets help with weight control—they literally feed your L cells the cues to keep you full.

It's worth noting that GLP-1 isn't the only incretin—a type of gut hormone that signals your pancreas to release insulin after you eat. Your upper small intestine houses K cells that secrete glucose-dependent insulinotropic polypeptide (GIP), the other major incretin hormone that helps boost insulin after meals. But GIP doesn't blunt appetite like GLP-1 and PYY do—it's more of a blood sugar specialist. GLP-1 has stolen the spotlight because of its dual role: managing glucose and reducing hunger.

The Colon's Niche: Slow Flow, Low Oxygen, Big Impact

The environment where these L cells operate is just as important as the cells themselves. By the time food reaches your colon, its movement has slowed to a crawl. In the small intestine, food usually clears out within a few hours, but in the colon, it can remain for thirty to forty hours. The prolonged contact means L cells get a sustained "dose" of whatever chemicals are in the mix.

And what a mix it is! As we know, the colon is an oxygen-free chamber packed with trillions of bacteria perfectly adapted to life without air. Those microbes are hard at work fermenting dietary fiber and resistant starches into Gut Gems that fuel your colon cells and signal to L cells. Moreover, the bile acids that weren't absorbed upstream are transformed by the colon into new forms. Some of these bile acids can activate receptors on L cells, adding another layer of hormonal stimulation. In short, the colon is a chemical reactor where microbial by-products can directly influence gut-hormone release.

Bacterial "GLP-1 Agonists" Akker's Proteins in Action

It turns out that Akker doesn't just influence gut hormones indirectly—it may directly trigger L cells through specific proteins. Scientists have begun isolating individual molecules from Akker to see what they do, and two star players have emerged so far: P9 and Amuc_1409.

These are Akker's secret weapons, with preclinical studies showing that Amuc_1409 regulates intestinal stem cells and supports epithelial homeostasis. P9 binds to intercellular adhesion molecule 2 (ICAM-2), a protein normally found on the surface of endothelial and immune cells that helps white blood cells stick to and move across blood vessel walls. ICAM-2 is also present on L cells; when P9 attaches to it, the result is GLP-1 release. When researchers purified P9 and gave it to diabetic mice, the result was elevated GLP-1 levels, reduced blood sugar, and increased burning of brown fat tissue, the metabolically active fat that generates heat and helps regulate body weight. This underlines a bigger point: Akker produces a toolbox of proteins that send positive messages to your body.

These bacterial proteins operate in a similar way to drugs, but in a gentler, more targeted fashion. P9, for instance, is essentially a microbial GLP-1 agonist akin to Ozempic and Wegovy. The difference is that it works by coaxing your own cells to release GLP-1. That means far fewer side effects, since it acts locally rather than flooding your whole system.

The mechanisms by which these proteins work likely involve immune signals. In experiments, mice missing the inflammatory signal IL-6 (an immune cytokine) did not respond to P9's glucose-improving effects, suggesting that the immune system plays a role. You can imagine the therapeutic potential: Purified postbiotic proteins from Akker could be developed as supplements to tap into the GLP-1 pathway naturally.

> 📌 **Gut Concept: P9**
>
> - **What it is:** P9 is a protein found on the surface of *Akkermansia muciniphila* (Akker), similar to Amuc_1100.
> - **Why it matters:** P9 acts like a signaling molecule, binding to receptors on host cells that influence immune balance and metabolism. Early research shows P9 can trigger the release of GLP-1, one of the key satiety hormones, and help fine-tune blood sugar regulation.
> - **How it works:** Even when Akker cells are pasteurized (heat-killed), some proteins remain active. P9 remains intact on their surface. In essence, P9 stimulates the L cell pathway as if a meal had arrived.

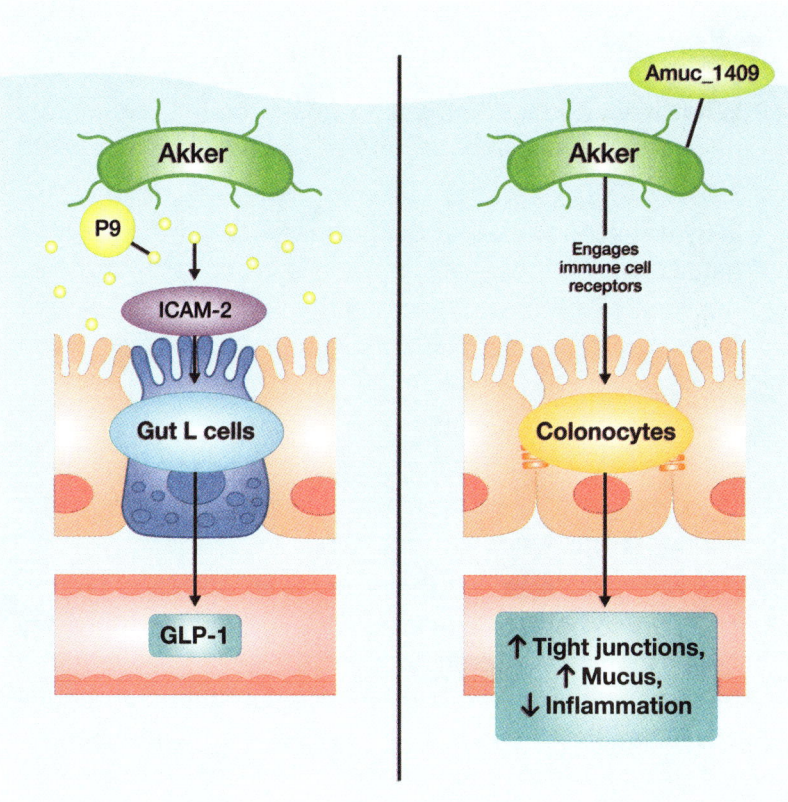

Figure 56. Akker's secret weapons: P9 binds ICAM-2 on L cells to trigger GLP-1 release, while Amuc_1409 acts on colonocytes to strengthen the intestinal barrier (tight junctions), promotes goblet cell differentiation indicative of increased mucus production, and mediates anti-inflammatory effects through immunomodulation, as shown in preclinical models.

- **Big picture:** P9 is one of Akker's molecular calling cards—a small surface protein with outsized influence. It helps explain why even pasteurized Akker delivers benefits, because its proteins keep signaling to your gut and metabolism even if the microbe itself isn't alive.

> 📌 **Gut Concept: Amuc_1409**
>
> - **What it is:** Amuc_1409 is a surface protein produced by *Akkermansia muciniphila* (Akker), alongside Amuc_1100 and P9.
> - **Why it matters:** Early evidence suggests that Amuc_1409 helps regulate intestinal stem cells and supports epithelial renewal, which may strengthen the gut barrier. Like other Akker proteins, Amuc_1409 may remain active even when the bacterium itself is dead.
> - **How it works:** Amuc_1409 sends a "renew and repair" signal to intestinal stem cells, prompting them to regenerate the gut lining. This renewal helps maintain barrier strength and overall gut balance.
> - **Big picture:** Together, these proteins sketch a postbiotic path to better gut health. What's exciting is that they operate much like drugs but in a gentler, more targeted fashion. The evidence is promising but still under active investigation.

Gut-Derived GLP-1 Versus Injections: Gentle Nudge or Giant Shove?

If Akker and its buddies can boost GLP-1, isn't that basically nature's version of a GLP-1 drug? Yes and no. Medications such as Ozempic act like a fire hose: They flood your body with a stable GLP-1 mimic, leading to dramatically higher hormone levels than normal. This massive activation of the GLP-1 receptor brings big benefits, as people can lose 15 percent of their body weight or more on these drugs.

The downside is that they often cause side effects such as nausea, vomiting, and altered taste, because so many GLP-1 receptors across the body are overstimulated at once. The endogenous GLP-1 you get from your L cells, by contrast, is

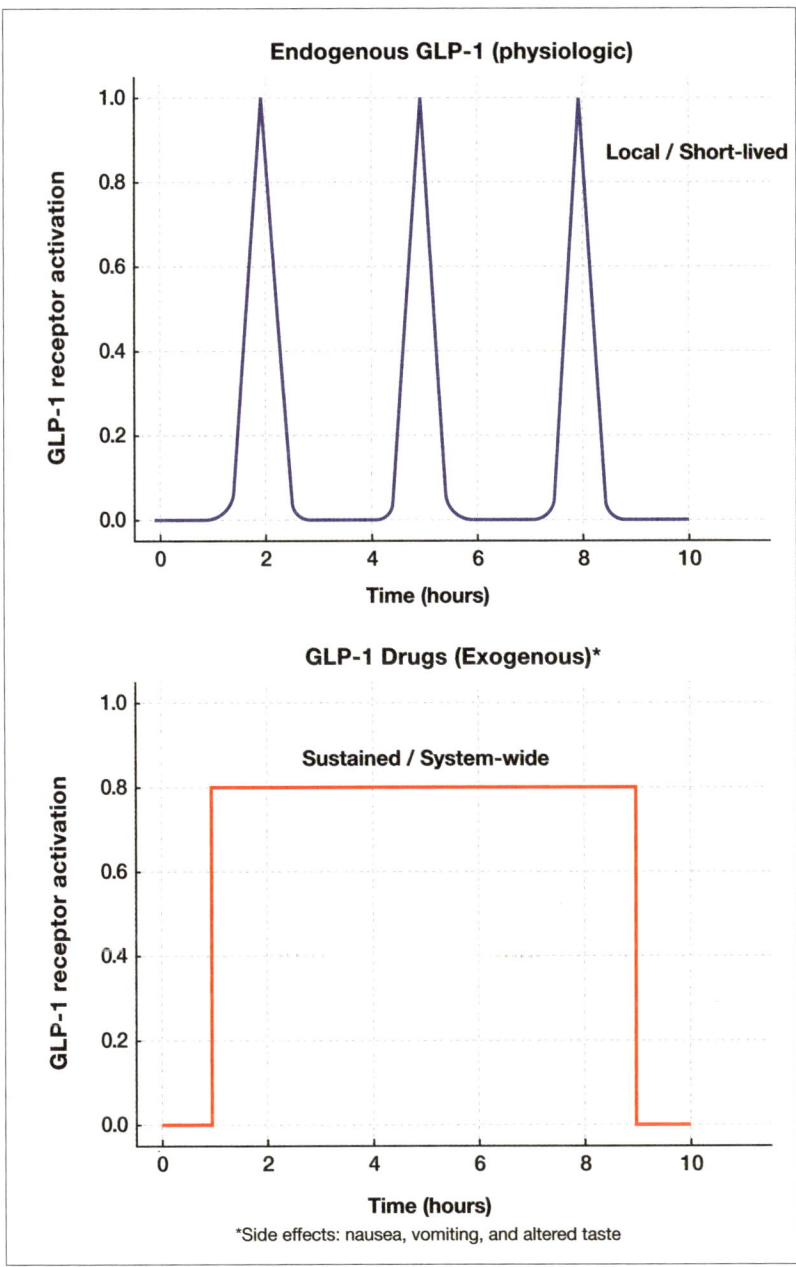

Figure 57. Endogenous GLP-1 is released in short, meal-triggered pulses, while GLP-1 drugs sustain prolonged receptor activation, explaining their stronger side effects.

more of a gentle nudge. In other words, your gut's GLP-1 is a short-acting local hormone, not meant to circulate at high levels system-wide for long.

These physiologic nudges won't melt fifty pounds by themselves. That's why experts suggest combining Akker with a diet low in fragile fats along with protein-forward meals, fiber, walking, and resistance training. Early studies confirm the efficacy of this combination. For example, volunteers taking pasteurized Akker for a few months saw improvements in insulin sensitivity and a slight drop in weight, but nothing like the jaw-dropping results of potent GLP-1 injections.

If you're looking to fine-tune metabolism and appetite over the long haul with minimal side effects, leveraging your gut's own GLP-1 system makes sense. By working with your body's natural signals, you're unlikely to overshoot to the point of nausea and more serious side effects, and your body will adjust meal by meal. One could imagine future protocols where a gut-targeted therapy, such as a postbiotic pill derived from Akker proteins, is paired with a very serious dietary commitment—specifically getting seed oils down to just 2 to 3 grams per day. This combination could amplify benefits while avoiding the side effects that come with GLP-1 drugs.

Early Evidence: Weight, Sugar, and Gut-Health Benefits

While all of this sounds great in theory—what about real-world results? The evidence, while still early, is encouraging. In mice, the benefits of Akker were noticed more than a decade ago: Obese mice given daily Akker ended up leaner, with less body fat and better glucose control than untreated mice. Their insulin resistance, and even fat-tissue inflammation, reversed to healthier levels, hinting that this microbe was doing something right inside the gut.

Follow-up studies in rodents reinforced these findings. For example, mice on high-fat diets showed thicker mucus layers and lower markers of gut leakiness and inflammation when supplemented with Akker—meaning fewer endotoxins, such as LPS from harmful bacteria, sneaking into their bloodstream. There's also evidence of bile acid remodeling: In animal models, Akker treatment shifted bile acid profiles in a way that ramped up metabolism. All told, rodent models have linked Akker to reduced weight gain, improved insulin sensitivity, stronger gut-barrier function, and lowered systemic inflammation.

Human data are more limited but starting to catch up. A landmark proof-of-concept study in Belgium recruited overweight and obese adults with insulin resistance and gave them pasteurized Akker supplements for three months. Compared to the placebo group, the Akker-supplemented participants saw significant improvements in insulin sensitivity—nearly 30 percent better on a lab index—and a drop in circulating insulin

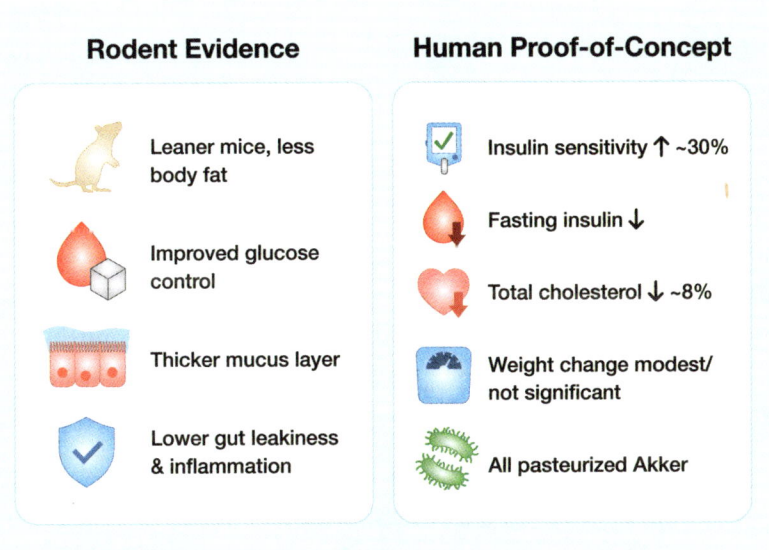

Figure 58. Evidence snapshot: Rodent studies show that Akker improves glucose control, mucus, and barrier integrity, while the human proof-of-concept trial demonstrated better insulin sensitivity, lower insulin and cholesterol, and modest weight change.

levels, suggesting their bodies were handling blood sugar more efficiently. Their total cholesterol also fell by about 8 percent, and inflammatory markers in the liver improved. Still, most findings beyond this Belgian trial come from preclinical animal research, so the human evidence base remains much thinner.

Beyond formal trials, researchers have consistently observed that people with healthier metabolic profiles tend to harbor more Akker in their guts. High Akker abundance has been correlated with leanness, better blood sugar regulation, and a more robust gut lining, whereas low levels are often seen in individuals with obesity, type 2 diabetes, or gut inflammation. These correlations align with the intervention studies. There are even hints that Akker may influence liver health by reducing fat buildup and shifting the body's overall inflammatory tone toward a healthier state. All of this has made Akker a celebrity in the microbiome world—one of the first next-generation probiotics to move from correlation to actual clinical testing. While larger and longer studies in humans are needed, the clinical signal so far suggests that boosting Akker or its key components can nudge multiple facets of metabolic health in the right direction.

Your Game Plan: Nurturing Akker and Amplifying GLP-1 Naturally

Ready to put this into action? Building a gut-friendly, hormone-boosting routine can be surprisingly straightforward. Here's a step-by-step game plan:

- **Boost Akker (probiotic or postbiotic).** Akker supplements are just starting to hit the market. In Europe, pasteurized Akker is authorized as a novel food, and supplements containing Akker—live or pasteurized—are already available. (And no, you won't find Akker in yogurt, kombucha, or other fermented foods since it doesn't survive in air.) However, new targeted microencapsulation formulas could provide that in the near future. Alternatively, you can try to raise your own Akker levels through diet (more on that next). The goal is simply to ensure this mucin-loving microbe is present in your gut in good numbers, either by adding it directly or encouraging its growth.

- **Feed the gut: prebiotics for mucus and Gut Gems.** Remember, Akker thrives on mucus—so you want to support your gut's mucus production and provide plenty of fermentable fiber for your microbiome. Make prebiotic-rich foods a daily part of your diet. Great options include inulin-rich foods such as chicory root, Jerusalem artichokes, and onions; resistant starches such as green bananas and rice or potatoes that have been cooked and cooled; and polyphenol-loaded foods such as cranberries, pomegranates, and red grapes.

- **Build a protein-forward diet.** Don't skimp on protein, especially at breakfast and lunch. High-protein meals are proven to increase GLP-1 and PYY release. Lean proteins such as fish, chicken, and Greek yogurt are great. A protein-forward diet not only helps with satiety but provides building blocks for maintaining muscle. If your main goal is weight loss, emphasizing protein (and fiber) will help curb cravings between meals. If your focus is blood sugar control, lean protein helps prevent glucose spikes after carb-heavy meals.

- **Add resistance training.** If there's a "magic pill" for weight loss, exercise is it. To increase GLP-1, resistance training is particularly beneficial. Lifting weights or doing bodyweight exercises builds muscle that soaks up glucose like a sponge. Plus, muscle contractions release IL-6, an exercise hormone that intriguingly prompts L cells to ramp up GLP-1 secretion.

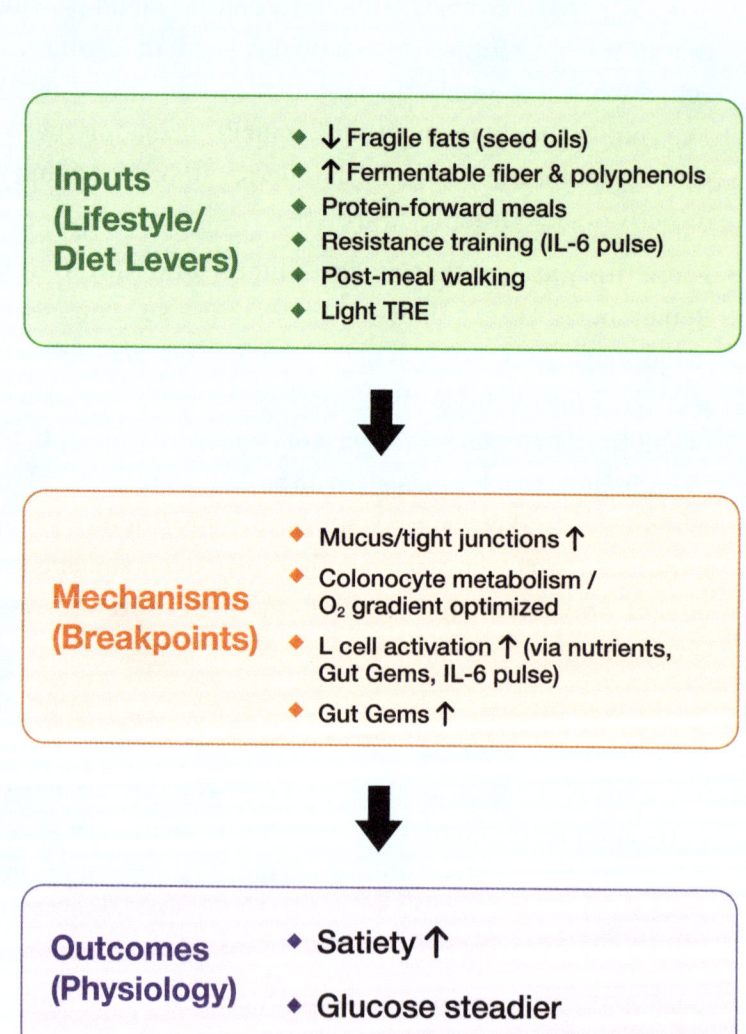

Figure 59. Lifestyle inputs (diet, exercise, timing) strengthen mucus, repair the barrier, and enhance L cell signals, leading to greater satiety and steadier glucose.

> 📌 **Gut Concept: Mercola Labs**
>
> - **What it is:** This is a built-in feature of the Mercola Health Coach app designed to guide your progress with customized fitness coaching and at-home lab testing.
> - **Mercola Labs:** This feature lets you track critical health markers from the comfort of home—like insulin resistance, inflammation, blood lipids, iron status, and hormone levels. The results give you objective proof of whether your plan is working. These tests cost up to 90 percent less than traditional labs and are done on your schedule, without the hassle of clinic visits.

Scan this QR code to get FREE access to the Mercola Health Coach app. This tool allows you to log your meals, track your macronutrient ratios, and monitor your progress over time.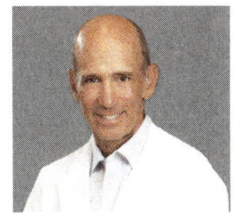

Finally, remember that everyone's biology is unique. Some people's guts will flourish with Akker through a few diet tweaks; others might need a probiotic to assist. Likewise, listen to your body: If increasing fiber causes discomfort at first, ramp up slowly and stay hydrated.

This isn't a one-size-fits-all prescription but a framework. If your main goal is fat loss, focus a bit more on regulating appetite through increased protein intake. If it's insulin sensitivity, prioritize exercise and fasting glucose metrics. You're essentially crafting a personal "gut-metabolic" program, so feel free to experiment and note what helps you most. Over time, these habits can synergistically tilt your biology toward a leaner, healthier, more energized you.

Weight-Loss Conquest: Your Victory Checkpoint

Today's 3-point scorecard:

1. **Tune in to satiety.** After each meal, rate your fullness from 1 to 10. This will help you tune in to what satiety feels like.

2. **Walk thirty to sixty minutes daily.** Low-intensity movement after meals blunts glucose spikes and reinforces satiety. Add a ten-to-fifteen-minute walk after each meal.

3. **Practice light TRE (time-restricted eating).** Aim for a simple twelve-to-fourteen-hour overnight fast; finish dinner earlier and breakfast a little later. This approach is an appetite "reset," not a punishment.

CHAPTER 7
How Dead Probiotics Help You Lose Weight

In previous chapters, we've discussed postbiotics and how even dead bacteria—the right kind of dead bacteria—can provide real benefits. In this chapter we'll do a deep dive into exactly how they work and what that means for your health.

Probiotic literally means "for life," suggesting a microbe must be alive to do good. Postbiotics flip that idea by providing all the benefits of probiotics but without the live bacteria. They're the harmless bacterial components that can still signal our bodies in positive ways. Postbiotics use components of friendly bacteria to nudge your body in the right direction. Your body recognizes certain molecular "fingerprints" on the dead bacteria or its fragments and treats them as allies, triggering effects such as a stronger gut barrier, reduced inflammation, and improved metabolism.

Unlike live probiotics, postbiotics don't have to survive the hostile trip through stomach acid; they can get to work immediately. Formally, scientists define a postbiotic as a preparation of inanimate microorganisms or their components that confers a health benefit. By this definition, a heat-killed probiotic pill full of cell fragments and metabolites counts as a postbiotic—and so does a filtered fermentation broth rich in vitamins and Gut Gems. The common thread is bioactivity without live bacteria.

Postbiotics have practical advantages over probiotics. Without needing to keep bacteria alive, products are more stable, require no refrigeration, and pose no worries about microbes dying on the shelf. They're also safer. Even people with weak immune systems or "leaky gut" can take postbiotics with minimal risk, because dead microbes can't overgrow or cause infections. Manufacturing is easier to standardize. And from a regulatory standpoint, using an inactivated microbe is simpler, since it's treated as a food ingredient or supplement rather than a live organism. In short, postbiotics offer many of the same perks as probiotics but in a more predictable, robust package.

Another big insight from postbiotics is that you can get benefits without establishing a live colony in your gut. Traditional probiotics aim to temporarily take up residence in your intestines to do their job, like houseguests who tidy up while they stay. Postbiotics, on the other hand, act more like a postal service, delivering messages and moving on. Even if your gut isn't welcoming to new bacterial tenants, you can still send signals to your body by mailing in these microbial "postcards."

Pasteurized Akker: A Postbiotic That Works Even When Dead

We've talked about Akker and its status as a rising star in gut and metabolic health research. Remember that Akker, when alive, helps maintain the mucus lining of your gut and communicates with your immune cells. Here's the twist: Scientists discovered that if you heat-kill Akker—essentially pasteurizing it, like milk—the dead bacteria can provide equal or even greater benefits compared to the live version.

Let's break down what happens when Akker is pasteurized. Although heating it renders it unable to grow or divide, its bacterial cells remain largely intact—picture an empty shell with important surface structures still in place. Akker also naturally releases tiny lipid bubbles called extracellular vesicles (EVs).

These are molecular messengers that microbes send out to communicate. Pasteurization doesn't destroy all of them; many survive the heating process, still packed with signaling molecules.

Akker's EVs can travel through the mucus layer and interact with cells in the gut, including hormone-producing cells. In animal studies, Akker EVs prompted these gut cells to release GLP-1 and PYY. In other words, the EVs act as mail carriers delivering messages such as "Tighten up the junctions between gut cells" (strengthening your gut barrier and repairing the leaks in the lining of your gut) or "Hey, release a bit more GLP-1 to help with that blood sugar spike."

> ### 📌 Gut Concept: EVs
>
> - **Full name:** Extracellular vesicles
> - **What they are:** EVs are tiny lipid "bubbles" naturally released by microbes such as *Akkermansia muciniphila* (Akker). Each vesicle is packed with proteins, lipids, and signaling molecules that can influence your gut and immune cells.
> - **Why they matter:** Even when Akker is pasteurized (heat-killed), many EVs remain intact. These vesicles can slip through the mucus layer and act as molecular messengers, delivering instructions to gut cells. In animal studies, Akker EVs boosted GLP-1 and PYY.
> - **What they do:** EVs deliver messages like "Tighten up those junctions" or "Release a bit more GLP-1." They provide another way pasteurized Akker can still deliver benefits.
> - **Big picture:** Think of EVs as microscopic mail carriers. They dispatch targeted letters from friendly microbes to your body's cells, nudging metabolism, appetite, and gut integrity in the right direction.

A small landmark trial tested daily capsules of Akker in overweight adults for three months. One group received live bacteria, another got pasteurized (dead) bacteria, and the control group got a placebo. The results put pasteurized Akker squarely in the spotlight. The group taking the dead bacteria saw a roughly 30 percent improvement in insulin sensitivity, meaning their bodies responded to insulin much better than before. Their fasting insulin levels dropped by about one-third, and their total cholesterol fell by around 9 percent.

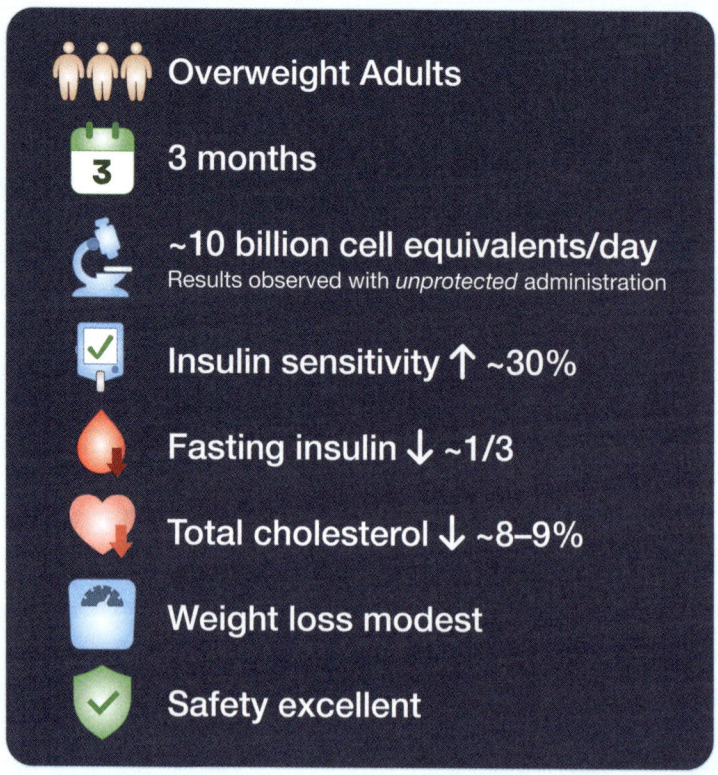

Figure 60. Summary of a small human trial showing pasteurized Akker improved insulin sensitivity and lowered insulin and cholesterol.

How Dead Probiotics Help You Lose Weight

Curiously, the group that got live Akker didn't show the same degree of benefit—the dead bacteria outperformed the live ones. This suggests that something about the pasteurization process might unlock or concentrate certain beneficial factors. Or perhaps the live Akker just didn't survive well through the digestive tract, so it couldn't do as much—a delivery problem we'll touch on later.

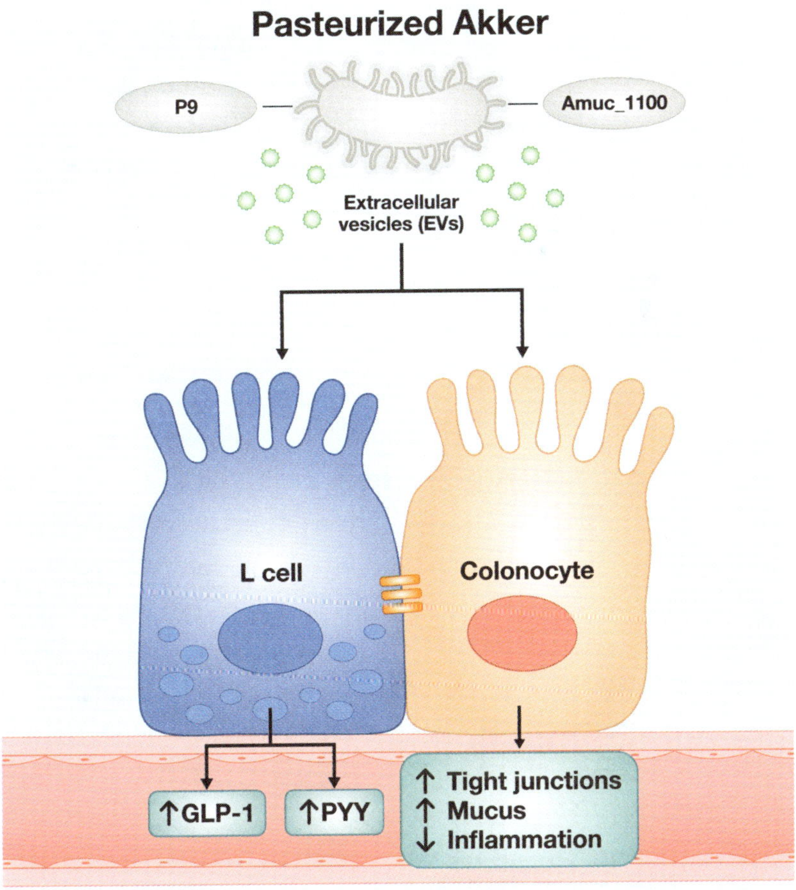

Figure 61. Pasteurized Akker signals via surface proteins and extracellular vesicles to boost gut-barrier function and hormone release.

Participants in the pasteurized group lost four to five pounds over three months, while participants in the live bacteria group lost about two pounds; the placebo group didn't lose any weight. The weight changes weren't large enough to be statistically relevant, but the trend favored the pasteurized postbiotic. Importantly, there were signs of a stronger gut barrier in the postbiotic group: Blood markers of "leaky gut" and inflammation, such as endotoxin levels and certain liver enzymes, improved only in those taking the pasteurized Akker. Still, it's worth a quick reality check. These trial results are exciting, but they don't guarantee the same outcome for everyone. Your gut, diet, stress load, and even sleep patterns all play a role in how postbiotics land. Think of this study as proof that the strategy *can* work, not a promise that it *will* work the same way in your body.

How Do Postbiotics Work?

Now that we've seen postbiotics in action, let's unpack how these dead microbes and their products actually do their jobs.

Structural Components (Proteins and Cell-Wall Pieces)— "Keys" That Unlock Healthy Responses

Bacterial cells are covered in unique patterns—think of them as molecular barcodes—that our bodies can detect. Even when a bacterium is dead, these structures, proteins, sugars, and bits of cell walls stick around. Our cells have special receptors always on the lookout for microbial patterns. When a postbiotic containing bacterial fragments comes along, those receptors bind to the pieces.

But because these signals come from a friendly source, they trigger a mild, beneficial activation instead of a full-blown alarm (as they do with GLP-1 agonists, such as Ozempic and Wegovy). For example, recall Akker's surface protein Amuc_1100. When it binds to TLR2 on gut cells, it sets off a chain reaction that strengthens the connections between gut-lining cells and boosts mucus production. In simple terms, the gut lining becomes tighter and better lubricated, creating a stronger barrier that keeps harmful substances out of your bloodstream.

Amazingly, certain postbiotic signals can turn on AMP-activated protein kinase (AMPK), a protein inside your cells that is sometimes called a master switch of metabolism. When AMPK is switched on, your cells burn more fat and use glucose more efficiently. It's also activated by exercise and intermittent fasting.

> ### 📌 Gut Concept: AMPK
>
> - **Full name:** adenosine monophosphate-activated protein kinase
> - **What it is:** AMPK is a protein inside your cells that functions as an energy regulator. It senses when cellular fuel is low and flips on pathways to restore balance.
> - **Why it matters:** When AMPK is activated, cells burn more fat, use glucose more efficiently, and improve insulin sensitivity. It's often called the master switch of metabolism. Exercise, time-restricted eating (TRE), and even certain postbiotic signals from your microbes can all flip this switch.
> - **Big picture:** Think of AMPK as your body's metabolic thermostat. When it switches on, it tells your system to clean up, burn fuel smarter, and restore energy balance, showing how lifestyle habits like TRE and gut-driven postbiotic signals work together to optimize metabolism.

Extracellular Vesicles—Microbial Mail Carriers

As mentioned earlier, many beneficial bacteria release tiny lipid bubbles filled with cargo, known as EVs. These vesicles can travel farther and slip through defenses more easily than whole cells. Postbiotic preparations often include these naturally produced EVs. In the context of metabolism, EVs from probiotics have been shown to act on the hormone-releasing cells in the gut.

EVs can carry all sorts of molecular cargo—proteins, lipids, and even bits of DNA or RNA—that influence your cells. Some

EV contents can dial down inflammation or reinforce the gut barrier. Interestingly, because EVs are basically little pieces of bacterial membrane, they carry some of the same molecular patterns that can engage our receptors from the inside. While a whole dead bacterium might only affect the cell it touches, that bacterium's EVs can spread out and deliver messages to cells farther away or even to other organs. This helps explain how consuming a postbiotic could lead to positive body-wide effects, such as improved insulin sensitivity.

Metabolites—Small Chemical Tools That Tune Our Metabolism and Immunity

While the first two mechanisms involve the physical components of bacteria, metabolites are tiny molecules produced

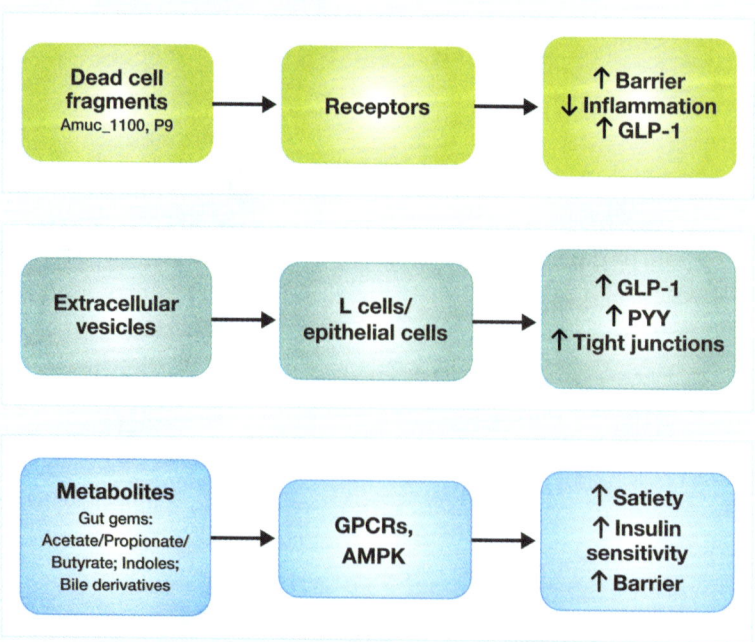

Figure 62. Dead cell fragments, extracellular vesicles, and metabolites act on host receptors to improve barrier function, reduce inflammation, enhance satiety, and boost insulin sensitivity.

during fermentation and other processes. If you've smelled fresh yogurt or sauerkraut, you've encountered bacterial metabolites. In our context, many metabolites made by gut microbes have beneficial effects, and they can either be included in a postbiotic product or produced in your gut when you feed your microbes certain foods. A classic example is the Gut Gem butyrate, which can activate AMPK and encourage metabolic flexibility. The following flowchart illustrates these mechanisms:

Acid, Bile, and Oxygen—Your Microbes' Worst Nightmare

Most people assume that if a bacterium is dead, its shell proteins just coast through digestion and show up in the colon untouched. Wrong. Your digestive tract is basically a biohazard obstacle course for fragile microbes, including the proteins from dead bacteria. This is because proteins, whether from food or postbiotic capsules, get pounded by acid, bile salts, and enzymes at every stage. Lab tests simulating digestion—first with pepsin, then with trypsin—show only a trace of intact protein remains by the end of digestion. The survivors become peptides before they reach the colon.

Without protection, the odds of delicate proteins such as P9 and Amuc_1100 making it through intact are virtually zero. Your stomach, with a pH hovering around 1–2, is as acidic as car battery acid. That's enough to destroy the function of most proteins and expose them to pepsin, an enzyme that cuts them into little peptide scraps. That means in the stomach alone, more than 99 percent of the intact protein is chopped up.

Survive the stomach? Great—now meet the small intestine's welcoming committee: bile and pancreatic enzymes. Bile is like a natural detergent—it breaks down fats in your food, but it also pokes holes in bacterial membranes, like a soap destroying grease. Then the pancreatic enzymes, especially proteases, join the party. These enzymes act like microscopic Pac-Men, chomping up proteins indiscriminately. So, if your pill contains a beneficial protein, say P9, and it somehow made it past the stomach acid, the pancreatic proteases might still slice it up before it gets anywhere.

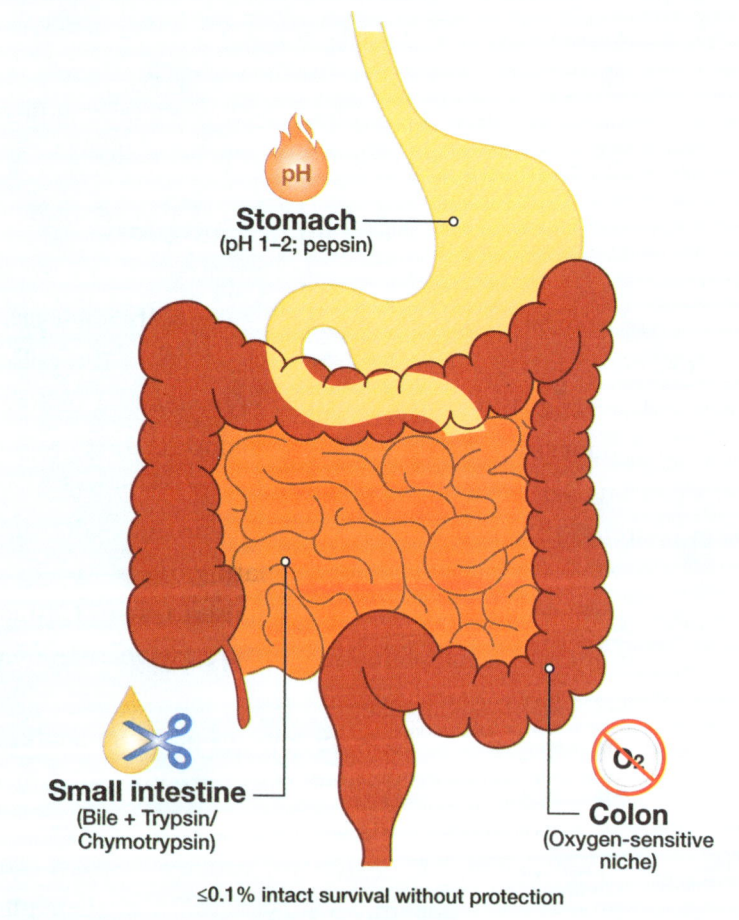

Figure 63. The digestive gauntlet: stomach acid, bile, enzymes, and an oxygen-sensitive colon challenge postbiotic survival.

In short, the digestive tract presents a gauntlet for anything you swallow: chemical destruction by acid and bile; enzymatic shredding; and the stealth killer, oxygen. No wonder getting probiotics or novel oral therapies to work is so tricky! To beat these barriers, we need some clever tricks up our sleeve.

A Double-Shield Breakthrough—Synthetic "Spores" and Glucomannan Fiber

If you can shield these proteins long enough for them to make it through the acid and enzyme gauntlet, you can dramatically amplify their impact. In this case, the technology needs to be tailored for live or pasteurized bacteria with fragile protein surfaces.

Fortunately, nature offers clues. Certain bacteria, like *Clostridium butyricum*, endure harsh conditions by forming spores: tough, seedlike packages built to withstand acid, heat, and even time itself. Most probiotic bacteria can't form spores naturally, but what if an artificial spore-like casing could be created for them? This synthetic spore doesn't "wake up" or release its cargo until conditions are just right.

Enter glucomannan: a natural fiber from the konjac root. Wrapped around the synthetic spore, glucomannan protects it from stomach acid and bile. Since humans don't make enzymes that can digest glucomannan, it stays intact throughout your stomach and small intestine, where the enzyme mannanase is able to crack it open. That means the protective shell dissolves only when the package reaches its destination—the colon.

The benefits don't stop at precision delivery. As glucomannan breaks down, it doubles as food for your resident microbes, giving the local flora a snack at the same moment the therapeutic payload—whether probiotics, postbiotics, or enzymes—breaks free in the colon. This allows your system to multitask—protecting, releasing, and nourishing all at once.

Protected by Our Global Patent—Your Gut Won't See This Anywhere Else

Companies, ours included, are racing to build delivery systems like the glucomannan synthetic spore. Ours is the only version protected by a global patent, ensuring this technology can't be replicated elsewhere. It's the only approach designed to

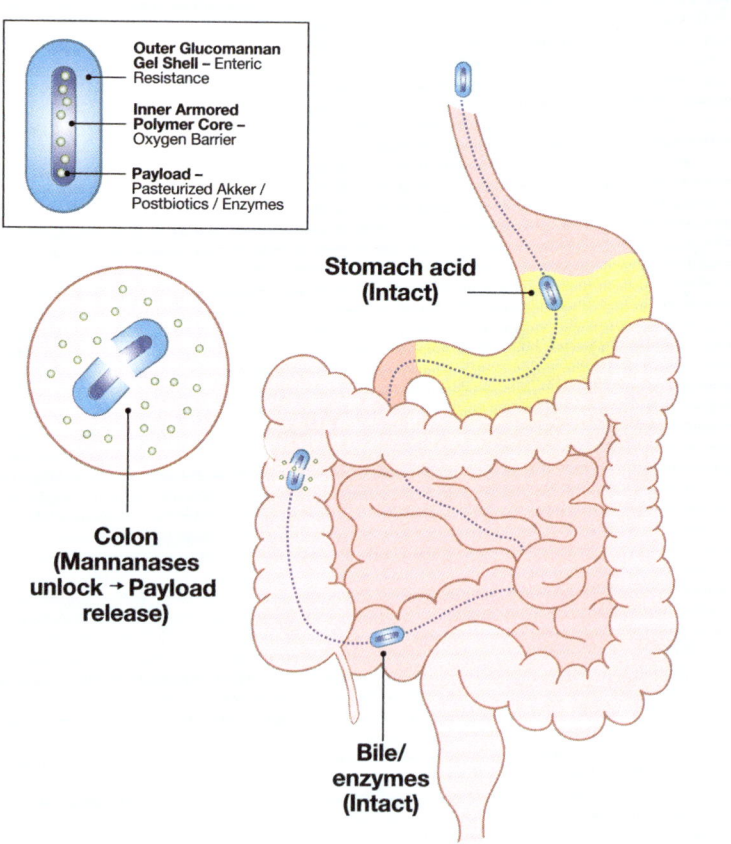

Figure 64. Cross-section of the double-shield capsule showing a glucomannan outer shell and polymer core protecting the payload until colon release

guarantee that intact proteins—not just fragments—reach the colon. Encapsulation within the polymer shell ensures safety, and glucomannan is a well-established dietary fiber. The mechanism is elegant: resistant in the upper gut and selectively unlocked by enzymes in the colon. In other words, it's a way to finally get fragile bacterial proteins through the gut gauntlet—dead but functional. It's the difference between releasing fragile seedlings in a storm versus planting them in a greenhouse and unveiling them only when the soil is ready.

Proving It Works: Simulated Guts, Stress Tests, and Survival Stats

This all sounds great—but how do we know they actually work? First, researchers put these delivery systems through a battery of tests: They get dunked in fake stomach acid, tossed into oxygen-rich environments, and more. Here are some of the ways we gauge success: In the lab, scientists can simulate the microbes' journey through the GI tract. They expose the capsule to simulated gastric fluid for, say, thirty to sixty minutes (the amount of time it would take to break down in the stomach), then expose it to simulated, higher-pH intestinal fluid with bile salts. Throughout the process, they check whether the capsule stays intact, only releasing at the right time. Researchers might use dye tracers or even real bacteria in these tests. If a capsule starts leaking or breaks too early in the acid phase, it's back to the drawing board!

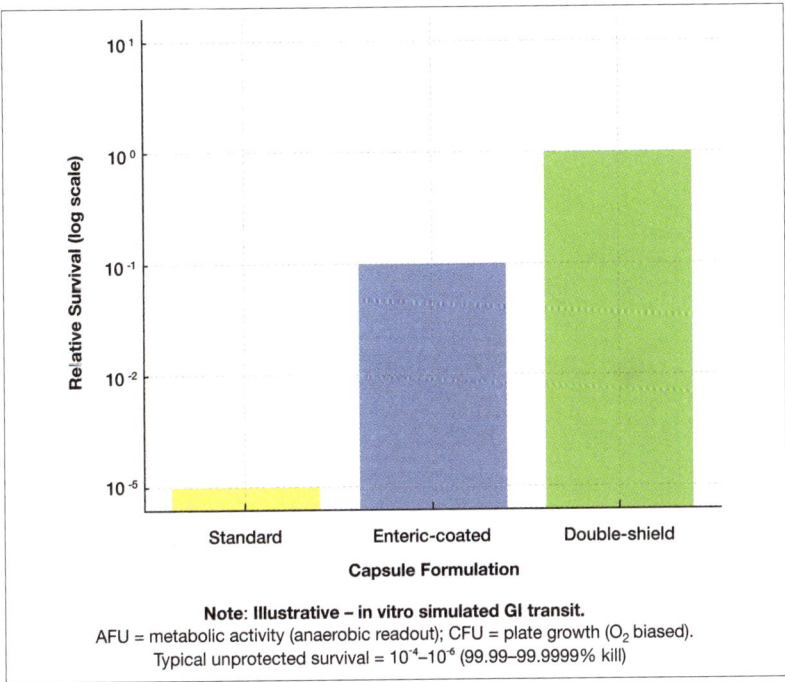

Note: Illustrative – in vitro simulated GI transit.
AFU = metabolic activity (anaerobic readout); CFU = plate growth (O_2 biased).
Typical unprotected survival = 10^{-4}–10^{-6} (99.99–99.9999% kill).

Figure 65. Relative survival of probiotics in simulated GI transit: Standard capsules show minimal survival, enteric coatings protect moderately, and double-shield design maintains the highest survival rate.

143

For oxygen-sensitive products, testers also examine how well the encapsulation protects against air. This might mean storing capsules in normal atmospheric conditions for a period and measuring how many bacteria survive versus identical capsules stored in an oxygen-free environment. A good anaerobic capsule should show high survival even when exposed to a small amount of oxygen. If unprotected capsules lose, for example, 90 percent of their bacteria after a day of air exposure, while protected ones lose only 10 percent, that's a huge win.

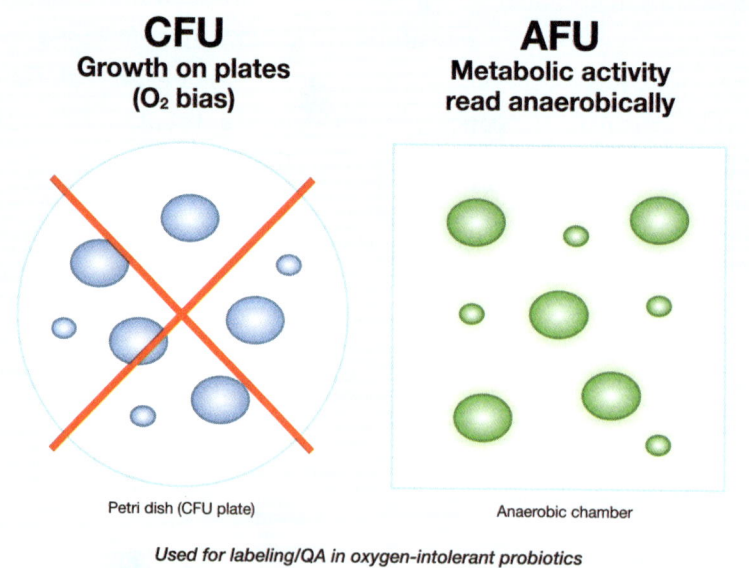

Figure 66. Comparison of CFU versus AFU methods for anaerobic viability. CFUs underestimate survival due to oxygen bias, while AFUs measure true metabolic activity anaerobically.

When it comes to oxygen-intolerant bacteria, the old way of counting survivors with colony-forming units (CFUs) doesn't really tell the full story. CFUs only work if the microbes can grow on a plate, which requires oxygen—exactly the condition these bacteria can't tolerate. That's why a different yardstick has become the norm: active fluorescent units (AFUs). AFUs don't rely on growth in oxygen; instead, they measure metabolic activity directly under anaerobic conditions, giving a more accurate read on how many microbes are truly viable. In fact, AFUs have become increasingly used for quality control of oxygen-sensitive probiotics such as Akker because they measure viable cells more inclusively than CFUs.

How to Use Postbiotics in Your Routine

A practical way to think of postbiotics is as one part of a gut health or wellness plan. Many experts suggest integrating postbiotics with other interventions for maximum effect.

Step 1: Repair Your Gut (Postbiotics First)

In the initial phase, your goal is to stabilize and repair your gut environment. If your gut barrier is leaky or your immune system is on high alert, it can be hard for other interventions (such as adding large amounts of fiber or new live bacteria) to take hold without causing discomfort. Postbiotics can act as first responders, quickly reinforcing the intestinal barrier and sending anti-inflammatory signals. For example, taking pasteurized Akker or a well-chosen postbiotic blend for a month or two could help restore your mucous layer and tighten the junctions between gut-lining cells, thereby reducing the leakage of endotoxins into your bloodstream.

Many people report that after a course of gut-targeted postbiotics, they experience less bloating and digestive upset. Make this stage count with two simple amplifiers: swap high-LA seed oils for butter, ghee, tallow, or coconut oil; and go for a ten-minute walk after meals. Both directly favor Akker's comeback.

During this period, it's also wise to eat a gentle, gut-friendly diet and to avoid irritants such as alcohol or NSAIDs (e.g., ibuprofen), which could counteract the healing process.

Step 2: Rebuild and Reinforce (Add Prebiotics, Then Probiotics If Needed)

Once you've done some repair, you can move to the next phase: nourishing your gut microbiome and adding new, living microbes. This is where prebiotics come in. Prebiotics are fermentable fibers or polyphenols that feed your good gut bacteria. Remember that dumping a load of fiber into an inflamed or imbalanced gut could cause a feeding frenzy of the wrong bacteria, leading to bloating, gas, and discomfort.

After step 1, however, you've improved the context: Your gut environment is less hostile, and your beneficial microbes have a better foothold. So, at this stage you can begin to gradually add prebiotics—such as inulin, FOS (fructooligosaccharides), resistant starch, or other fiber supplements. These help foster the growth of the right microbes. If you want, you can also add a probiotic at this stage, to supply new, live microbes.

Pay attention to how you feel day to day: Are your energy levels better? Fewer afternoon sugar crashes? Are cravings for sweets decreasing? These subjective clues are important, too. For gut health specifically, you could track your digestion and stool habits. Simply noting changes like "less bloating," "more regular bowel movements," or improvements in stool consistency can tell you a lot. If your bloating has gone down and your bathroom trips are more comfortable, it's a sign your gut barrier and microbiome are in a better place than before. By sequencing this way—repair → rebuild → reinforce—you avoid overwhelming your system. Postbiotics shine in that initial repair stage. Prebiotics and probiotics then build on that groundwork to cultivate a lasting healthy ecosystem in your gut. This layered approach can be more effective than doing these strategies alone.

Another benefit of this step-by-step approach is that you can tell which step triggers symptoms and adjust accordingly. Over time, you'll discover the right maintenance routine for you. That might mean continuing a low dose of a postbiotic for ongoing support; keeping plenty of prebiotic foods in your daily diet; and cycling through different probiotics for variety, if you choose. The following diagram shows in detail how this two-stage plan works.

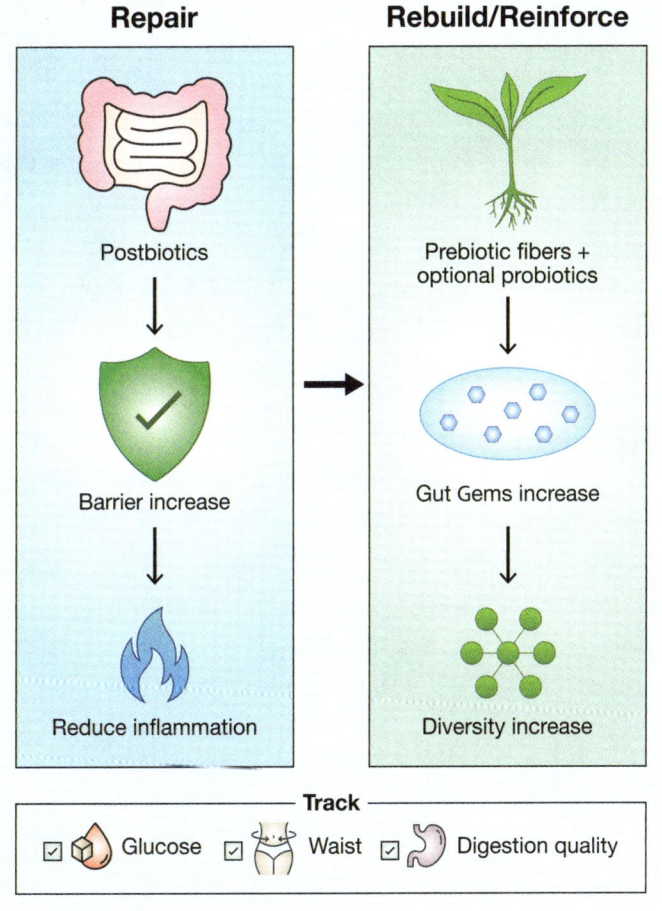

Figure 67. Two-stage road map: First, postbiotics repair the gut barrier, then prebiotics and probiotics rebuild diversity.

Remember, maintaining improvements is an ongoing process. You'll likely want to continue with a balanced diet rich in prebiotic fibers—plenty of veggies, some fruit, whole grains, and legumes; add a postbiotic a few times a week (or daily if it makes you feel noticeably better); and maintain a gut-friendly lifestyle by managing stress, getting enough sleep, and staying active. Postbiotics are simply another tool in your wellness kit.

Your Three-Step Postbiotic Plan

To wrap things up, here's a simple three-step action plan for introducing postbiotics into your routine.

Step 1: Power Up with Postbiotics

Pick one postbiotic supplement or food to incorporate and see how you feel. For example, you might try a pasteurized Akker capsule or even a postbiotic-rich fermented product (some supplements provide just the broth, which is full of metabolites).

Action: Add it to your daily routine for a few weeks and note any changes in digestion, energy, or cravings.

Step 2: Support Your Gut Lining

Identify a couple of simple habits that strengthen your gut barrier. For instance, swap out alcohol for a gut-friendly alternative such as kombucha or herbal tea, or add a fiber supplement or a fiber-rich snack to feed your mucus-building microbes. Probiotics can also be used.

Action: Choose one of these habits and start today.

Step 3: Track Your Progress

Check in regularly—ideally daily—with the Mercola Health Coach app to stay accountable, especially for diet and exercise changes that counteract the damage from seed oils and poor habits.

Action: Inside the app, choose one health metric that matters most to you—waist circumference, fasting blood sugar, energy levels, or even how often you feel bloated—and monitor it over time. Over a month or two, you'll see the changes: a smaller waist, consistently lower glucose, and more sustained energy throughout the day. Each improvement is a win, and the Health Coach app will celebrate them with you! By following a plan like this, you're actively shaping your health journey—adding something new, supporting it with good habits, and tracking how it helps you. Over time, you'll be able to determine what kind of impact postbiotics have for you and how they best fit into your lifestyle.

 Scan this QR code to get FREE access to the Mercola Health Coach app. This tool allows you to log your meals, track your macronutrient ratios, and monitor your progress over time.

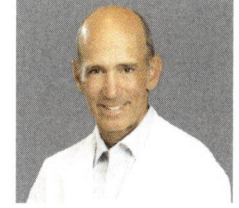

CHAPTER 8
The Fiber Paradox

As you learned in chapters 1 and 4, fiber is an essential component of gut health. Not all bacteria need the same type of fiber, however. The microbes in your gut have different food preferences. Some species love the gel-like fiber in oats; others, the crunchy cellulose in veggies. By offering a rainbow of fibers, you support a broader range of helpful microbes.

This is called functional redundancy, and it's like having backup players on a team. If one microbe has an off day, another steps in to keep producing vital nutrients. This diversity also sets the stage for Akker to flourish. The result is a more resilient gut ecosystem.

Some fibers break down quickly in the upper colon, while others travel farther to feed microbes in the lower gut. This staggered breakdown ensures no section of your colon goes unfed. Without variety, parts of your microbial community could starve. In fact, a consistently fiber-poor diet can cause helpful species to dwindle. By rotating foods containing different fiber types, you create a safety net. Different microbes produce overlapping enzymes to digest fiber; when many species share the workload, the system flourishes. That fiber-fueled stability makes a difference in how you feel day to day. A diverse fiber intake is linked to more consistent digestion (fewer swings between constipation and diarrhea) and even-keeled metabolism.

You might notice steadier energy and fewer crazy hunger pangs when your gut community is balanced. A varied, high-fiber diet keeps your gut calm. You don't need a weekly shot to blunt your appetite because fermentation nudges your own GLP-1 and PYY production. Remember that these peacekeeper microbes only thrive in an oxygen-free zone. Fiber fermentation helps them in two ways: It makes them grow, and it produces acids that lower gut pH, ensuring a suitable environment. By contrast, a diet lacking fiber diversity allows oxygen and pH levels to creep up, inviting less friendly, typically disease-causing bacteria and yeasts to settle in.

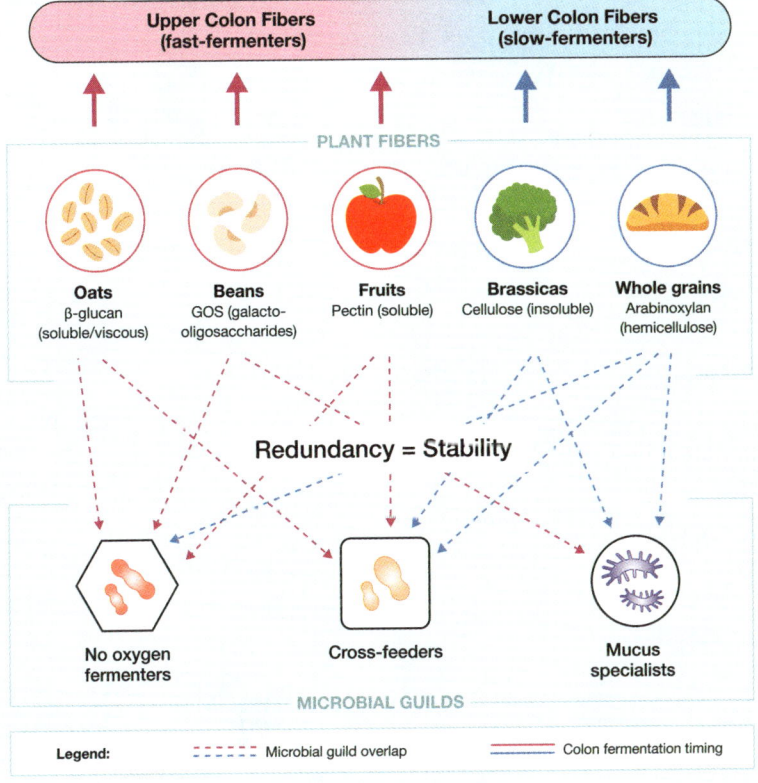

Figure 68. Diverse plant fibers feed overlapping microbial guilds across the colon, creating stability through functional redundancy.

Simple amplifiers multiply the effect: Walk ten to fifteen minutes after meals; swap seed oils for butter, ghee, coconut oil, or tallow; and rotate plant fibers through the week. Next time you plan a meal, imagine you're crafting a menu for the population of that diverse, bustling city.

Bottom line: Diversity in your diet breeds diversity in your gut, and that's the foundation of a resilient, health-boosting microbiome.

The Fiber Paradox: When a Damaged Gut Says "Not So Fast"

But what if your gut lining is inflamed and leaky? In this state, even the healthiest fiber can backfire. Instead of exclusively feeding friendly microbes, that load of fermentable fiber might also fuel the troublemakers.

One big culprit is lipopolysaccharide (LPS), a cell-wall component of certain bacteria. LPS binds to Toll-like receptor 4 (TLR4), a protein on immune cells that acts like a smoke detector for bacterial invaders. This binding triggers a release of pro-inflammatory cytokines, chemical messengers that scream "Inflammation!" The result is more damage to your gut lining and a ripple of inflammation through your body.

> 📌 **Gut Concept: TLR4**
>
> - **Full name:** Toll-like receptor 4
> - **What it is:** TLR4 is a receptor protein on the surface of immune cells. Its specialty is detecting LPS (endotoxin), a fragment shed by certain bacteria.
> - **Why it matters:** When LPS binds to TLR4, it's like a smoke detector going off. This alarm triggers immune cells to release inflammatory cytokines.
> - **Gut impact:** The cytokine surge ramps up inflammation, weakens your gut barrier, and can ripple outward

into whole-body problems such as insulin resistance and chronic inflammation.

- **Big picture:** Think of TLR4 as your immune system's fire alarm. It's essential for spotting real threats, but when leaky gut lets LPS slip through, the alarm gets pulled too often—putting your body in constant overdrive.

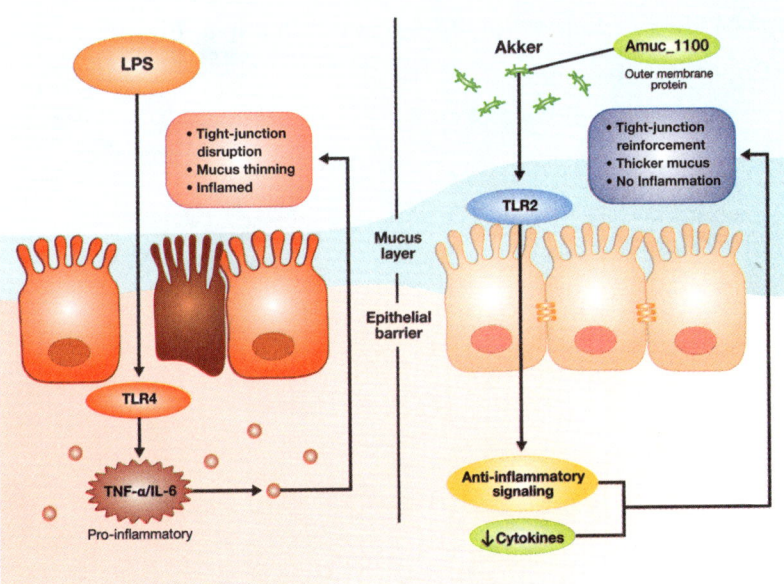

Figure 69. TLR4/LPS drives cytokines and leakiness, while TLR2/Amuc_1100 reinforces tight junctions and mucus.

It's a vicious cycle: Inflammation weakens your gut barrier, leading to more inflammation. Over time, you can develop chronic, low-grade metabolic inflammation—often linked to insulin resistance and stubborn weight gain. (If you've been struggling to lose weight despite eating "right," hidden gut inflammation could be part of the problem.) In extreme cases, a flood of LPS and bacteria hitting the bloodstream at once can lead to sepsis—a life-threatening whole-body inflammation. While rare (sepsis usually develops only in severe infections), it underscores how crucial it is to heal your gut barrier before you bombard it with tons of fermentable fiber.

The smart play is to go slow. Start with low-fermentability fibers and small portions. For example, you might begin with well-cooked, soft veggies such as carrots or peeled zucchini—fibers that are gentler and partially broken down—rather than a big raw kale salad or a chicory-root fiber supplement. Pay attention to how you feel. Fermented foods or a probiotic can help reintroduce good bacteria, but start those gradually, too.

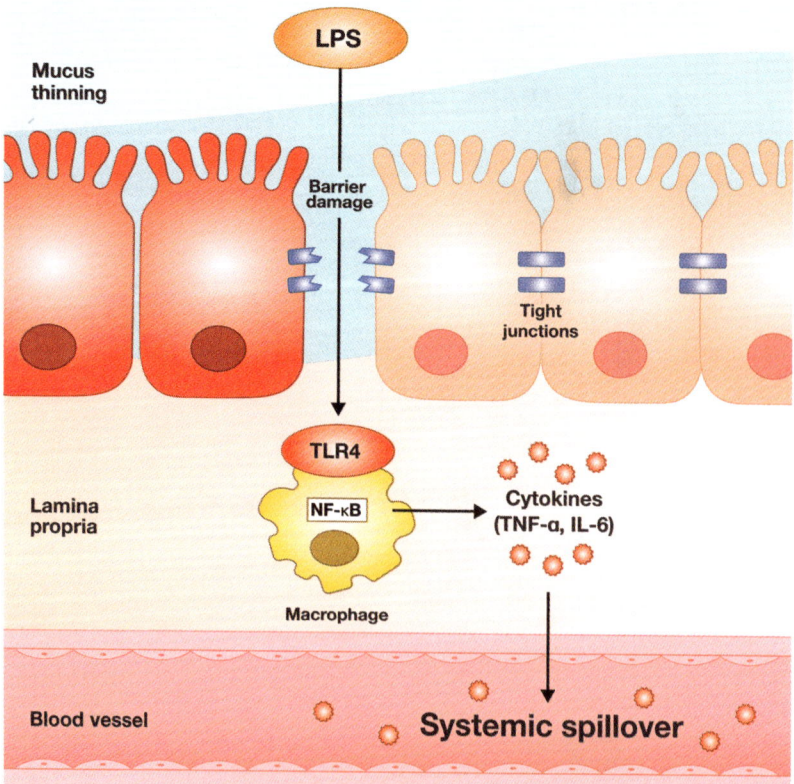

Figure 70. LPS crossing a weakened gut barrier activates TLR4, releasing cytokines and driving systemic spillover.

Keep in mind that fiber isn't the villain here—it all depends on context. As Akker rebounds and TLR2 signaling rises, tolerance usually improves, at which point you can gradually increase fiber again. Many people find that after a period of gut healing, foods that once caused bloating become much more tolerable. Patience is key. Add one new fiber-rich food at a time and give your system a few days to adjust. And don't forget hydration and gentle movement. Even short walks can help move things along comfortably.

Know Your Fiber Types and What They Do

The payoff isn't just "regularity." It's metabolic calm via natural GLP-1 signaling and a tighter barrier, which makes appetite-suppressing drugs redundant. Remember, not all fiber is created equal—different types act differently in your body.

- **Soluble/viscous fiber**—found in oats, beans, and fruit pectin—dissolves in water to a gel, slows sugar absorption, binds cholesterol-rich bile, and ferments into Gut Gems.
- **Insoluble fiber**—found in whole grains and veggie skins—does not dissolve, adds bulk to stool, speeds up transit, helps keep you regular, and ferments little so there's less gas.
- **Resistant starch**—found in cooled rice or potatoes and green bananas—escapes digestion, arrives intact in the colon, and is fermented by gut microbes into abundant butyrate.
- **Hemicellulose (arabinoxylan)**—found in whole grains such as rice bran—requires microbial teamwork to break down, yielding Gut Gems and bolstering the gut's mucus barrier.

Each type of fiber has its superpower. Soluble fiber, like the pectin in your apple or the beta-glucan in your oatmeal, is a champ at steadying blood sugar and lowering cholesterol. It forms a gel in your gut that slows how fast you absorb glucose and traps some fats along the way. Meanwhile, your microbes love soluble fiber. As they ferment it, they crank out Gut Gems that nourish your colon cells and tame inflammation.

Insoluble fiber, on the other hand, is the classic "roughage." Think of the stringy strands in celery or the bran flakes in your cereal. It doesn't turn into gel or dissolve—it just sweeps through your intestines, providing bulk and a scouring action that helps prevent constipation. Insoluble fiber basically exercises your gut muscles by giving them something solid to push against.

Then there's resistant starch—often dubbed the third type of fiber. This starch sneaks through your small intestine untouched, only to become a feast for bacteria in the colon. There are actually four subtypes (RS1, RS2, RS3, RS4), depending on the source and how the starch is prepared, but all of them share a resistance to digestion. What makes resistant starch special is its butyrate-boosting ability. When your microbes munch on resistant starch, they produce loads of butyrate—the superstar Gut Gem that feeds your colon lining, strengthens your gut barrier, and even supports metabolic health. People who include legumes and cooled starchy foods often notice improved digestion and satiety. Resistant starch also tends to be easier on the gut than some fiber (although individual tolerance still varies), so it's a great "training fiber" if you're still building up tolerance.

Finally, we have hemicellulose, a broad category of plant fiber, with arabinoxylan being a notable one in whole grains. It often needs multiple species of microbes to break it down. This cross-feeding means hemicellulose helps foster a cooperative, diverse microbiome. The payoff is a mix of Gut Gems and a boost to your gut's mucus layer. In fact, research suggests that arabinoxylan from wheat bran can improve intestinal barrier function, essentially making your gut lining tougher. So, while hemicellulose might not be as well-known as, say, psyllium, it quietly bolsters your gut health when you eat whole grains and veggies.

At the end of the day, a healthy diet means a mix of fiber. Variety ensures you reap all the benefits: smoother digestion, a well-fueled gut lining, better blood sugar control, and even bonus perks such as lower cholesterol and improved regularity. You don't have to plan fiber selection at every meal. By simply mixing up your plant foods, you'll naturally cover all the bases. Now you know why fiber isn't just fiber—it's a whole family of helpers on your plate!

Fiber and Polyphenols: A Gut-Health Dynamic Duo

Fiber has a powerful sidekick in polyphenols, colorful plant compounds in fruit, tea, coffee, cocoa, and spices. When you pair fiber with polyphenol-rich foods, you're essentially double-teaming your gut microbes with nutrition and bioactive signals. Polyphenols themselves aren't fiber—they're antioxidants and pigments—but they interact closely with your microbiome. For one, many polyphenols resist absorption, so they're able to make it to your colon, where your gut bugs get a chance to feast on them. Your microbes then break these complex plant chemicals into smaller metabolites that your body can actually use. Some of those metabolites (such as gut-derived urolithins from pomegranates) have anti-inflammatory and even anticancer properties, giving you benefits you wouldn't get from the original form of the polyphenol alone. It's a beautiful symbiosis: You give microbes polyphenols, and they turn them into health-promoting molecules.

But that's not all—polyphenols also shape who's in your microbial community. For example, the polyphenols in berries, red grapes, and green tea have been shown to inhibit some opportunistic bacteria while boosting friendly ones. This helps keep the microbiome balanced and the environment in the colon more hospitable for the good guys. Polyphenols also have antioxidant effects right there in the gut, soaking up excess free radicals.

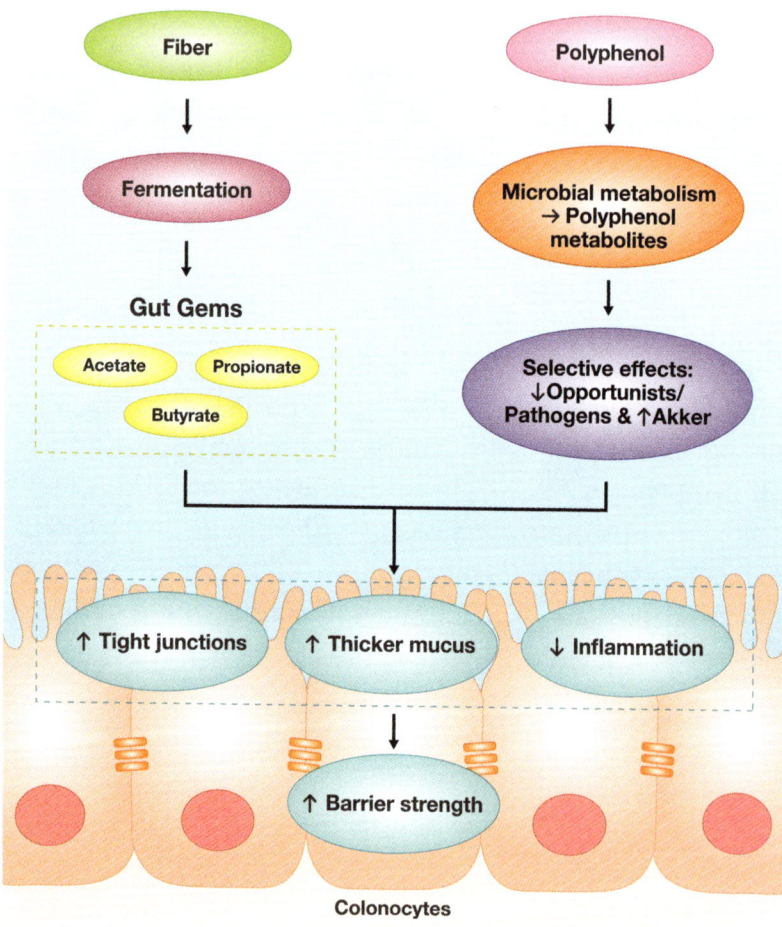

Figure 71. Fiber and polyphenols act through complementary microbial pathways to boost Gut Gems, support Akker, and reinforce the gut barrier.

It turns out certain polyphenols are like fertilizer for Akker. In research, mice given cranberry, grape, or pomegranate extracts (all rich in specific polyphenols) showed a blooming of their Akker populations. Scientists think this is because polyphenols reduce gut stress and inflammation, creating a comfy habitat for Akker; and with inflammation down, the gut makes more of the mucin that Akker feeds on. In human studies, diets high in polyphenols are associated with higher Akker levels and markers of better metabolic health.

Practically speaking, this fiber–polyphenol tag team is easy to harness. Nature already packages them together in many foods—an apple, for instance, contains soluble fiber and polyphenols in its skin. But you can also mix and match. Sprinkle cinnamon (rich in polyphenols) onto your high-fiber oatmeal. Have berries or a cup of green tea with your whole-grain toast. Add cocoa powder to a chia-seed pudding. These combinations make your gut bugs sing. Over time, with more beneficial metabolites circulating in your body, you may notice positive effects on your appetite and weight. It's amazing how a simple choice like adding color to your high-fiber meals can translate into tangible health payoffs.

The Fermentation Cascade: From Fiber to Fuel

When fiber finally reaches your colon, it kicks off a chain reaction of goodness. Picture a domino effect where each step creates a healthier environment for your gut. Here's the rundown of what happens when fiber ferments:

1. **Fiber fermentation begins.** Gut bacteria break down fiber and release Gut Gems.
2. **Gut lining is fed.** Butyrate fuels your colon cells, helping them repair and strengthen the gut barrier with tighter junctions and more protective mucus.
3. **pH drops, gut is happier.** Gut Gems make the colon slightly acidic, which helps friendly bacteria thrive while many pesky microbes struggle to cope.
4. **Oxygen levels fall.** Well-fed colon cells use up more oxygen, keeping your gut oxygen-free—just how your best microbes like it.

This positive feedback loop means that the more fiber your microbes get, the more they improve the habitat to favor even more good microbes. One extra perk: Those Gut Gems also signal your body to release appetite-regulating hormones. So, this fermentation not only nourishes your gut lining and blocks out invaders but also helps tune your metabolism and appetite from the inside out. That's a cascade worth cheering about!

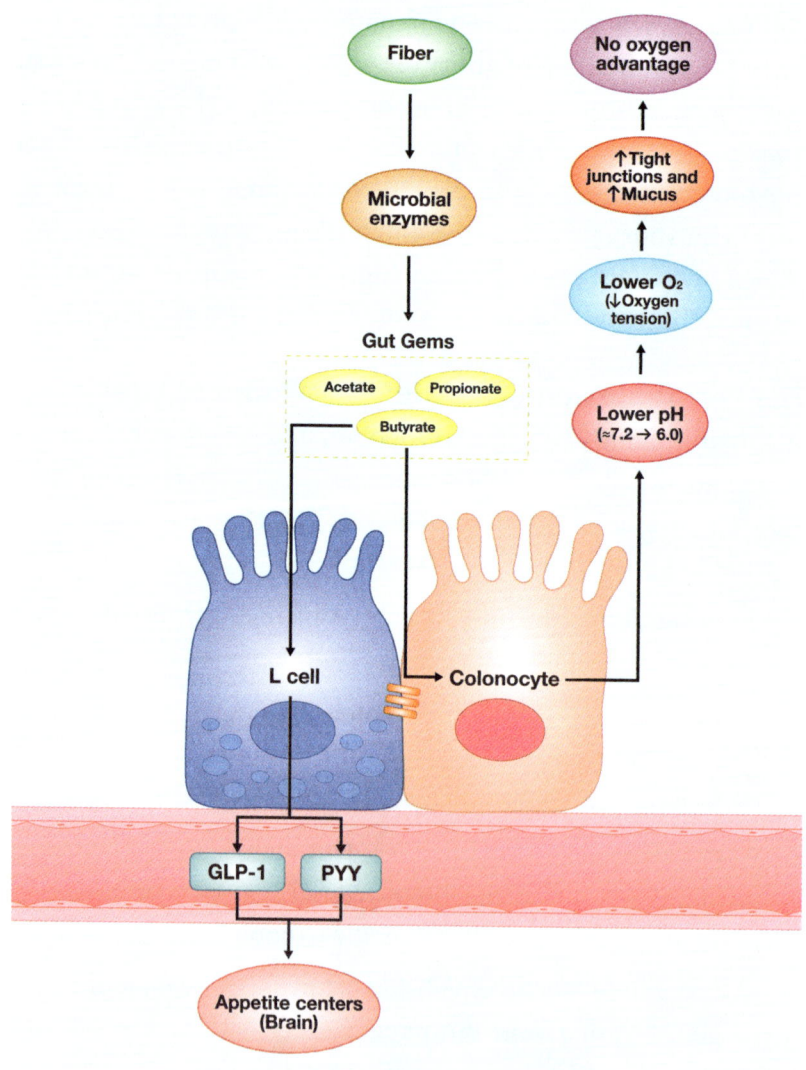

Figure 72. Fiber fermentation fuels colon cells (colonocytes), lowers pH/oxygen, strengthens the barrier, and boosts satiety hormones.

Pacing Your Fiber Upgrade: Slow and Steady Wins

Remembering that "slow and steady wins the race" can save you a lot of bellyaches. When starting to level up your fiber intake, choose wisely. Gentler types of fiber—such as cooked carrots, squashes, ripe bananas, or oats—tend to be well tolerated. As weeks go by and you slowly introduce diverse fiber, you'll likely find you can enjoy foods that previously made you bloat without issue. A tip during this build-up phase: hydrate, hydrate, hydrate. Fiber soaks up water like a sponge in your intestines—that's part of how it adds bulk and softens stool. But if you don't drink enough, that sponge can turn into a brick. Aim to drink a glass of water with each meal and throughout the day. Minerals like magnesium and potassium help your intestinal muscles contract normally, so they're your friends in keeping things moving as you increase fiber. And don't skimp on protein: Your gut-lining cells (colonocytes) need amino acids to regenerate, and protein at meals also helps you feel satisfied.

Finally, pay attention to your body's feedback. Tracking simple things—like bloating levels, stool consistency, or even morning fasting blood sugar—can tell you a lot about your progress. If you want objective proof, you can now order tests such as fasting glucose and hs-CRP, a sensitive marker of inflammation, directly through Mercola Labs inside the Health Coach app.

 Scan this QR code to get FREE access to the Mercola Health Coach app. This tool allows you to log your meals, track your macronutrient ratios, and monitor your progress over time.

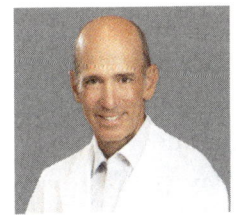

Many people find that as they increase fiber, their blood sugar readings stabilize and their CRP levels drop—clear signs that their gut and metabolism are moving in the right direction. Plus, your bathroom reports will tell you if you're hitting the sweet spot. If things get too loose or gassy, that's a sign to slow down and stay at that level a bit longer before pushing ahead. Remember, this isn't a one-week sprint; it's a lifestyle marathon.

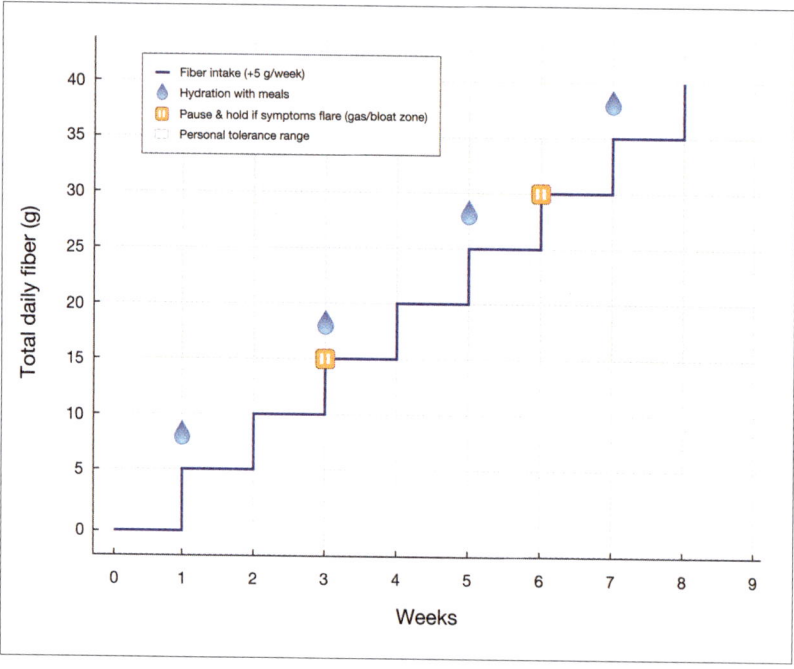

Figure 73. Gradual fiber increase with hydration cues, symptom pause points, and a 25–35 g/day target range

In Real Life: Your Daily Gut-Friendly Game Plan

So, to recap: Aim to rotate and combine different fiber sources throughout the week so you cover all your bases without getting bored. For example, start one morning with a warm bowl of oatmeal topped with blueberries (polyphenols galore). The next day, enjoy a protein-rich omelet with a side of sautéed mixed veggies. Have you heard of the potato salad trick? Chilling potatoes or rice cooked the day before dramatically increases their resistant starch content. Green bananas are another resistant starch bomb (try blending a small chunk of green banana or plantain into a smoothie).

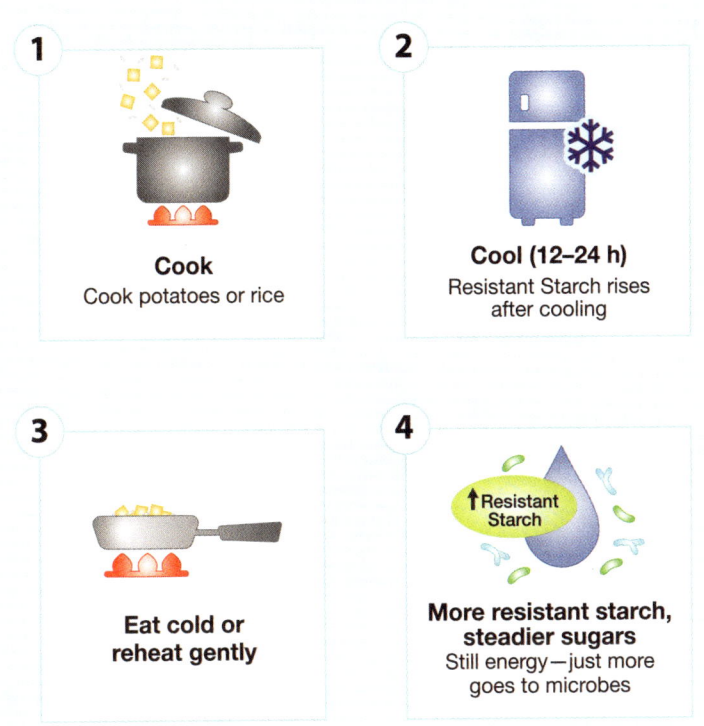

Figure 74. Cooking, cooling, and gently reheating starches such as potatoes or rice raises resistant starch, steadies blood sugar, and feeds gut microbes.

Don't forget the fruits and veggies! These are fiber-and-polyphenol double whammies, especially if you eat the peels/skins when possible. A skin-on apple or pear a day, berries, grapes, citrus, pomegranates—take your pick, you really can't go wrong. And try to get a serving of cruciferous veggies—broccoli, cabbage, brussels sprouts—most days. You can roast them, stir-fry them, or toss them into soups. Not only are they loaded with insoluble fiber but they also contain unique plant compounds that may aid in detoxing unwanted substances in your gut. Remember to pair fibers with polyphenols whenever you can. Have a cup of green tea or iced hibiscus tea with your lunch instead of soda. Snack on a few squares of dark chocolate in the afternoon. Season your food liberally with herbs and spices. These little add-ons not only make meals more delicious but also give an extra boost to your gut health. As you build your daily fiber habits, remember the golden rule: Prioritize variety and consistency over any single "superfood." Eating ten different plants a day beats eating ten servings of broccoli. By weaving fiber seamlessly into your routine, you'll soon notice it's just a natural part of your meals—and you'll be reaping the rewards in energy, mood, and yes, easier weight management thanks to that well-nourished GLP-1 factory in your belly. Just remember to introduce new fiber sources slowly, to avoid discomfort.

Fiber Cheat Sheet: A Quick Look at Types, Microbes, and Benefits

We've covered a lot of ground. Here's a handy snapshot of the major fiber classes, some key food sources, the gut all-stars they support (hello, Akker!), and the standout Gut Gems they tend to produce.

Fiber Class	Key Foods	Typical Serving (g fiber)	Gas Potential	Predominant Gut Gems	Notables
Soluble/ Viscous	Oats, Beans, Apples	4–6 g	Medium	Acetate, Propionate	Beta-glucan, Pectin
Insoluble	Whole grains, Veggie skins	2–4 g	Low	Minimal Gut Gems	Cellulose
Resistant Starch	Cooled potatoes, Green bananas	3–5 g	High	Butyrate	RS1–RS4
Hemicellulose	Whole grains, Rice bran	2–3 g	Medium	Mixed Gut Gems	Arabinoxylan

Mix for diversity; variety over volume.

Figure 75. Quick-reference table summarizing major fiber classes, key foods, serving sizes, gas potential, SCFAs, and special notes

Real-World Win: From Sluggish to Supercharged

Maria, a forty-five-year-old self-proclaimed junk-food lover, never imagined fiber could change her life. She started off exhausted, a bit overweight, and dealing with daily bloating. With a family history of colon polyps, her doctor gently suggested she boost her fiber intake for overall health. Maria was skeptical—could something as simple as veggies and whole grains make a difference?

She began small: swapping her usual sugary breakfast pastry for overnight oats with berries and nuts. The first week she felt a little gassy, but she persisted. Each week Maria added another fiber tweak: whole-grain bread instead of white, an apple as an afternoon snack, black bean chili. She sipped green tea with lunch instead of her usual cola. By the end of the month, she noticed she wasn't crashing at 3:00 p.m. anymore—her energy was steadier. And that pesky belly bloat was gone.

Fast-forward three months and Maria has lost eight pounds without "dieting." She attributes it to feeling fuller on fiber and ditching processed snacks. Her latest bloodwork showed a dip in fasting blood sugar and her hs-CRP dropped into the normal range. Maria's favorite change? "My sweet cravings disappeared," she laughs. Now she keeps a rainbow of foods in her fridge and enjoys mixing and matching fiber and polyphenols. "It's not a diet anymore; it's just how I eat," she says. And knowing she's likely slashing her colon cancer risk in the process is the cherry on top. In fact, she's now inspiring her family to join her fiber journey, proving that small daily changes can lead to big health payoffs.

Weight Loss Conquests: Your Victory Checkpoint

Today's 3-point scorecard:

1. **Diversify.** Add at least one new high-fiber food (fruit, veggie, or legume) to one meal today.

2. **Aim high (fiber).** Swap a low-fiber snack for a fiber-and-polyphenol combo (for example, an apple with dark chocolate).

3. **Hydrate.** Drink two extra glasses of water to keep your fiber routine running smoothly.

CHAPTER 9

A Two-Step Restoration Protocol

Think of your gut as a garden. You wouldn't scatter seeds on lifeless, dry soil and expect a lush harvest. First you'd enrich the soil and pull out the weeds. In the same way, our two-step restoration protocol works by repairing your gut's mucosal barrier *before* adding beneficial microbes. A sturdy mucosal barrier means any new friendly bacteria you introduce can actually settle in and do their job.

As we've discussed in previous chapters, when the barrier is compromised, toxic bacterial bits can slip into your bloodstream and overactivate your immune system. This chronic commotion can drive up inflammation, interfere with blood sugar regulation, and pack on stubborn weight around your belly.

So before tackling weight loss or metabolic health head-on, fix the foundation to create an environment where good microbes thrive. Step 1 is all about calming things down and patching up your gut's defenses. Step 2 adds targeted probiotics to keep those defenses strong and boost your metabolism naturally.

Many people pop probiotics like candy and wonder why they don't feel a difference. It's like tossing expensive fish into a polluted pond. Our two-step protocol ensures you clean the "pond" first. Only then do we introduce the star of the show:

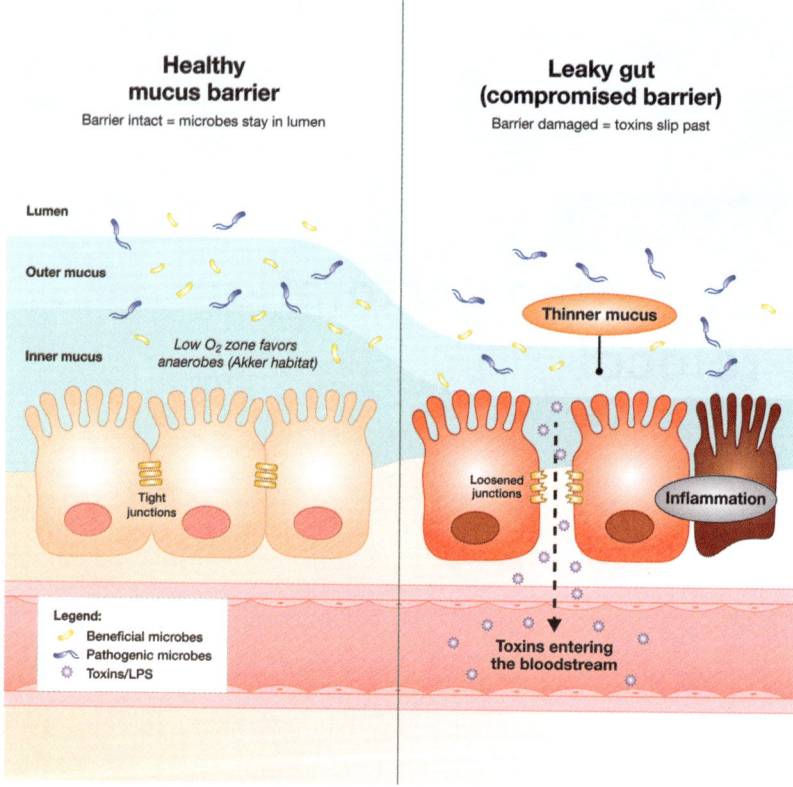

Figure 76. Repairing the gut barrier prevents toxin leakage, reduces inflammation, and prepares the habitat for beneficial microbes.

Akker, the rock star gut bacterium that can support your body's appetite-control and blood-sugar-balancing systems. Unlike most probiotics, Akker is a keystone species—think of it as the scaffolding that helps your gut community stay stable. When Akker shows up, the whole neighborhood functions better, which is why it gets special focus in this protocol.

In short, this chapter's protocol helps you harness your gut's natural powers in a logical sequence. By following this plan, you'll be nudging your body to produce more GLP-1 in a gentler way than the new injectables provide. Let's dive into phase 1.

A Two-Step Restoration Protocol

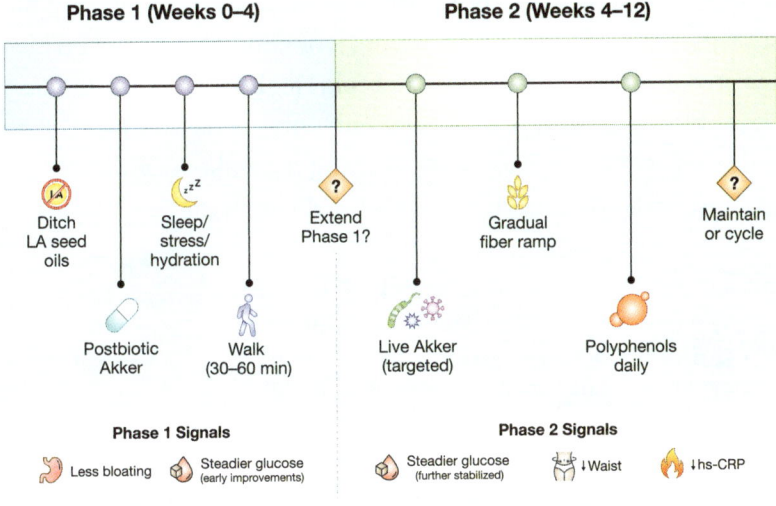

Figure 77. Twelve-week road map timeline showing phase 1 (repair) and phase 2 (reseeding), with actions, checkpoints, and markers of progress

Phase 1: Barrier Repair (Weeks 0–4)—Remove the Bad Fats, Add Gut-Healing Signals

It's time to roll up your sleeves for the first month. Phase 1 is all about reducing gut saboteurs and giving your belly a chance to heal. Over the next four weeks, your game plan has three parts:

1. Ditch inflammatory seed oils.
2. Take a daily Akker postbiotic supplement.
3. Nail the healthy-life basics: sleep, stress management, hydration, and gentle movement (aim for thirty to sixty minutes of walking daily).

Let's break those down.

Remove Inflammatory Fragile Fats in Seed Oils

As already made clear, industrial seed oils—basically the fats in most processed and fast foods—are sky-high in fragile fats. In excess, these act like gas on the fire of inflammation. Even worse, these oils can disrupt your gut flora and thin out that precious mucus barrier. You might be shocked that even "healthy" salad dressings or nut butters hide soybean or canola oil—but don't fret about reading labels. Our new Mercola Health Coach app makes it easier than ever to spot and eliminate dangerous fragile fats from your diet by identifying them, keeping a detailed record of food choices, and guiding you step-by-step through the process.

Scan this QR code to get FREE access to the Mercola Health Coach app. This tool allows you to log your meals, track your macronutrient ratios, and monitor your progress over time.

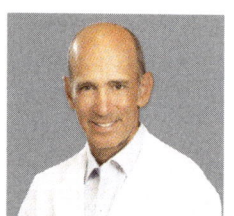

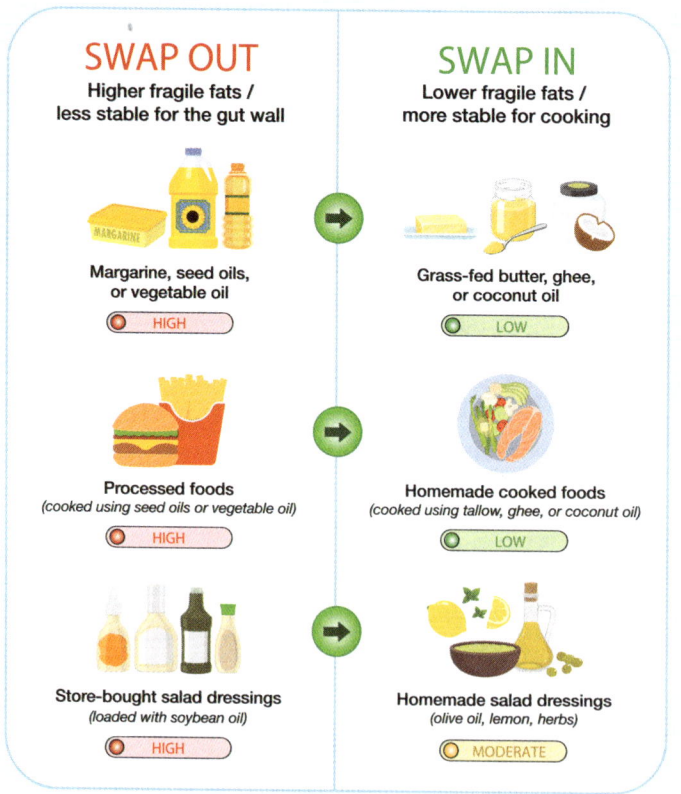

Figure 78. Cooking fats spectrum swap: Replace high-LA seed oils and processed foods with lower-LA, stable fats to support gut-barrier integrity.

Stock up on friendly fats such as coconut oil, grass-fed butter or ghee, and even beef tallow for high-heat cooking. These are far more stable, much lower in fragile fats, and won't wage war on your gut lining.

Take a Daily Postbiotic Akker Booster
Now we're going to send some "friendly signals" to your gut lining. Remember our superstar microbe, Akker? In phase 1, you'll take it as a postbiotic—that is, as pasteurized cells. Think of it as a practice run for the habitat.

Practical tip: Many cutting-edge gut supplements now include pasteurized Akker, sometimes labeled as "Akker postbiotic" or as part of an "afterbiotics" blend. Take one daily, ideally in the morning on an empty stomach.

Lock In the Lifestyle Basics
Lastly, phase 1 is the perfect time to get your healthy habits on track. Your gut can't heal if you're running on four hours of sleep and chronic stress. Think of these as nonnegotiable pillars of gut repair:

- **Sleep:** Aim for seven to eight hours per night, with a regular bedtime. Your intestinal cells do major repair work while you're snoozing.
- **Stress relief:** Find a de-stress method that works for you—whether deep breathing, short walks, yoga, journaling, or dancing in your kitchen—whatever lowers your cortisol.
- **Hydration:** Drink plenty of water and replenish your electrolytes (a pinch of mineral salt in water or an electrolyte drink). A well-hydrated mucosal layer is a happy one.
- **Gentle movement:** Keep it low intensity for now—think daily walks, stretching, or light yoga. Movement helps

your gut motility (keeps things moving along) and relieves stress, without the strain of intense exercise.

By the end of these four weeks, you should notice signs of progress, such as less bloating, more regular digestion. You may even shed a pound or two. Your gut will have a sturdier wall and be ready for the next phase. And remember, you can always extend this repair phase a bit longer until you're ready to move on. Assuming all lights are green, phase 2 awaits—time to reintroduce our microbial buddies!

Phase 2: Reseeding (Weeks 4–12)—Planting the Good Bugs for Lasting Metabolic Wins

With your gut barrier on the mend, it's time to reintroduce beneficial microbes to your ecosystem. The star here is live Akker—those mucus-loving "good bugs" we primed your gut for in phase 1. Over the next eight weeks (around weeks 4–12), you'll be adding probiotics in a targeted way to colonize your gut with the right helpers.

Add Live Akker (Targeted Delivery)
Adding live Akker as a probiotic is a bit trickier than tossing back your average yogurt culture. As mentioned, this bacterium hates oxygen, it's fragile, and in a plain capsule it would be destroyed by stomach acid long before ever reaching its real home in your colon. If you want to get live Akker to your colon, special technology is needed. Our targeted Akker is the only one in the world that can deliver nearly all of the bacteria alive, thanks to a patented glucomannan fiber "bubble shield" that doesn't break down until it reaches your colon. Because this system is protected by patent for the next nineteen years, no competitor can legally copy it. In short, other brands may give you some postbiotic benefit, but only this delivery system ensures you're getting the living keystone species right where it belongs.

A Two-Step Restoration Protocol

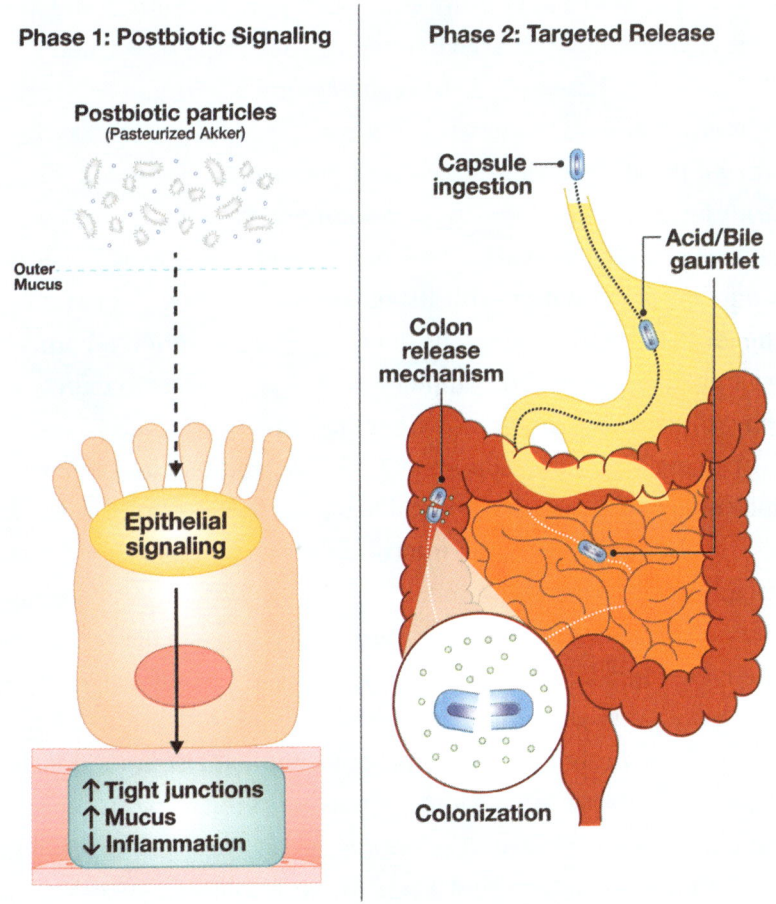

Figure 79. Two-step probiotic strategy: Postbiotic signaling strengthens the barrier; targeted capsule delivers live cells to the colon.

Consider Complementary Strains

While Akker is the headliner, you can bring in a couple of sidekicks in phase 2 for an even more robust gut community. The key is to choose noncompeting probiotics that won't elbow Akker out of its niche. One of the best strains to consider right away is *Clostridium butyricum*, another oxygen-intolerant microbe like Akker—and one of the very few that can reliably reach your colon alive because it naturally forms a protective spore. That spore acts as its own built-in armor, allowing it to survive digestion and arrive intact in your large intestine.

The catch, however, is that *Clostridium butyricum* needs the right environment to thrive once it gets there, which means supporting it with the right fibers and conditions. Some advanced formulations currently in development bundle Akker with helpers such as *Faecalibacterium prausnitzii*, a strong butyrate producer, along with carefully selected prebiotics. And looking ahead, our team is actively developing nine other advanced organisms designed to complement Akker, which we expect to bring to market within the next year.

During phase 2, keep an eye on how you feel as you introduce new probiotics. It's normal to have a day or two of mild gas or bowel changes as your microbiome shifts—that's just your gut adjusting to new residents. If anything feels off, such as significantly looser stools or cramping, you can scale back to every other day and build up slowly. By week 12, you'll have given your new gut bugs plenty of time to take root. Akker and friends should now be busily churning out beneficial compounds. In other words, your microbiome is now working *for* you, keeping hunger in check and blood sugar stable. Up next, let's talk about the fuel and cofactors that keep this microbiome-metabolism machine humming.

Fueling and Cofactors—Feed Your Gut Garden with Polyphenols and Fiber

As we discussed in the previous chapter, Akker and friends love fiber. But timing matters. Loading up on fiber too early can backfire. Once you're ready, fiber becomes a powerful ally. If your main goal is weight loss, emphasizing fiber helps keep you full on fewer calories. If your top priority is better blood sugar control, then the polyphenol-rich foods we discussed earlier—such as tea, berries, or cinnamon—can help steady glucose levels while also supporting your gut flora.

Load up on polyphenols. Remember that colorful polyphenols feed beneficial microbes, including Akker. Aim to incorporate polyphenol-rich foods daily: berries, cherries, red grapes, green or black tea, mycotoxin-free coffee, or dark chocolate are easy to work into a meal or have as a snack. Herbs and spices are polyphenol powerhouses too, so sprinkle cinnamon in yogurt or add oregano and turmeric to your cooking.

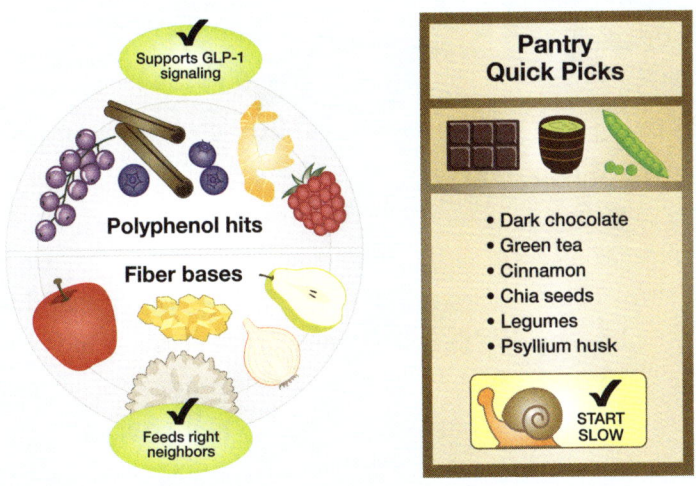

Figure 80. Plate and pantry map of gut-friendly foods showing polyphenol hits and fiber bases with quick picks and a "start slow" reminder

Fill up on fermentable fibers (slowly). If polyphenols are the metabolic boosters, fiber is the steady fuel for your gut bugs. Fibers such as resistant starch, pectin, inulin, beta-glucan, and arabinoxylan are basically breakfast, lunch, and dinner for your colon microbes. When bacteria chow down on these fibers, they produce Gut Gems that help heal your gut lining, reduce inflammation, and signal your brain that you're full. Here are some easy ways to add fiber:

- Add a small scoop of resistant starch to a smoothie (potato starch or green banana flour works well) or enjoy a half cup of cooked-then-cooled rice or potatoes. (Cooling forms resistant starch—a neat trick!)

- Include a daily serving of high-pectin fruit, such as an apple with the skin or some berries.

- Experiment with arabinoxylan-rich grains if you tolerate them: a bit of oats, barley, or a whole-grain cracker. If you're grain-free, consider a teaspoon of psyllium husk in water—it's mostly arabinoxylan fiber—but be sure to drink plenty of water with it.

Monitoring and Milestones—Tracking Progress and Knowing When to Pivot

To make sure this protocol is delivering results—and to know when to tweak something—you'll want to track a few key metrics. Think of these as your personal scorecard for gut and metabolic health. You don't need to check daily—weekly or biweekly is fine—but keep notes so you can spot trends. Here are three of the most important to track: weight, waist size, and body fat. Body weight and waist size are useful markers. Weigh yourself about once a week (at the same time of day) and measure your waist circumference (around your navel) every couple of weeks. A waist-to-height ratio below 0.5 is a good goal since it means your waist is less than half your height. If you start at 0.6 and work toward 0.55 or below, that's real progress, even if the scale isn't moving much. A shrinking waistline usually signals less visceral fat—the risky stuff packed around your organs that drives inflammation. But here's the thing: While waist and hip sizes are helpful, they're still rough guesses.

Fasting blood sugar and insulin: Use a home glucose meter or lab test to track your fasting glucose. Are you trending down toward the 80s or low 90s mg/dL? That's fantastic. If you can get a fasting insulin reading, even better: You can then calculate your HOMA-IR (an insulin resistance score). For example, an insulin level of 15 µIU/mL and glucose of 100 mg/dL gives a HOMA-IR of approximately 3.7, which is high; seeing that number drop closer to 1–2 over time would be a win. Don't stress if you can't test insulin—just know that improvements in fasting glucose, or a lower hemoglobin A1C (HbA1c) from your doctor, are clear signs your insulin sensitivity is improving.

Inflammation marker high-sensitivity C-reactive protein (hs-CRP): This one requires a lab test, but hs-CRP is one of the best gauges of overall inflammation. If your hs-CRP is high (above 3 mg/L is considered high risk), you'll want to see it drop closer to 1 or below. Many people notice their CRP falls as they lose weight and heal their gut. It's not something you need to measure often, but it's a smart checkpoint at the end of phase 2, if you can.

Digestion and stool monitoring: Tune in to how your digestive system feels. Are you less bloated than before? How's your stool consistency and frequency? Ideally you're having comfortable daily bowel movements that are medium-brown and well formed (not little rabbit pellets or loose water). The Bristol Stool Form Scale pegs ideal poop at types 3 and 4. Keep a simple journal: Note your energy levels, any digestive upset, and even mood or brain fog. The gut-brain axis is real—steadier energy and mood can be a sign your gut inflammation is down.

End of Phase 2 (Week 12): This is the big assessment. By now, you should notice significant shifts: You're not getting midafternoon energy crashes and that sweet tooth is less demanding. Check those metrics again: weight, waist measurement, and labs. This is the moment to decide on your next steps. Many people will be happy with the progress and transition into maintenance mode (continuing the healthy habits and maybe a lower maintenance dose of the probiotics). If you still have a ways to go to reach your goals, you can plan another cycle or integrate additional strategies.

WEIGHT LOSS CURE: MELT FAT NATURALLY

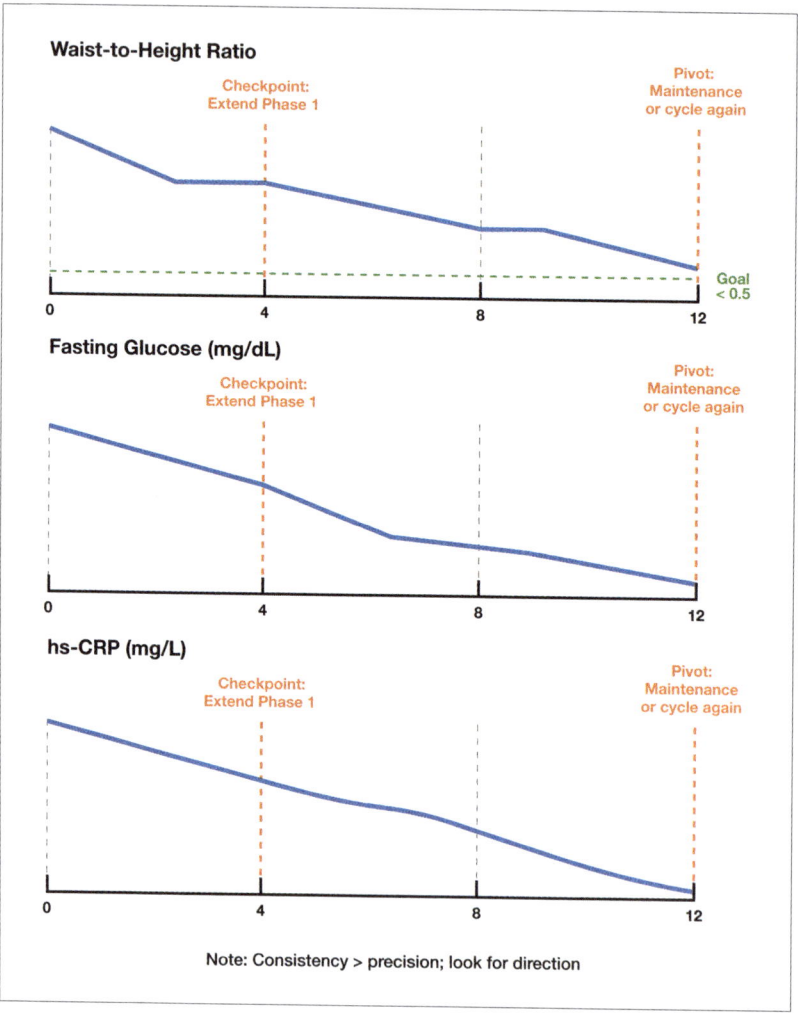

Figure 81. Sample progress chart with sparklines for waist-to-height ratio, fasting glucose, and hs-CRP over twelve weeks, with checkpoints at weeks 4 and week 12 and icons highlighting key health goals

Expected Outcomes—a Healthier, Happier You (What This Protocol Delivers)

By committing to this two-step restoration, you're setting the stage for some pretty awesome payoffs. They won't all happen overnight, but gradually you should experience:

- **Natural appetite control:** One of the first things many people notice is enhanced satiety. You may feel full sooner during meals, and those crazy cravings should diminish. This is your body responding to better GLP-1 signaling and stable blood sugar.

- **Steady weight loss:** With improved appetite regulation and less inflammation, your weight should trend downward at a sustainable pace. Maybe it's a pound a week, maybe more if you have a lot to lose. The key is, you're losing fat, not muscle, because you're not crash-dieting—you're nourishing yourself. Over twelve weeks, it's totally realistic to shed 5 percent or more of your body weight, which is clinically significant for health.

- **Better blood sugar control:** Expect lower fasting glucose and fewer energy swings. Many people report that the afternoon slump disappears—no more reaching for a latte or needing a nap at 3:00 p.m. If you started with prediabetes or insulin resistance, don't be surprised if your next labs show reduced risk for type 2 diabetes.

- **Reduced inflammation and pain:** As your gut barrier heals and those inflammatory signals calm down, you may notice improvements in seemingly unrelated areas—less joint pain, fewer breakouts, even eczema patches clearing. Systemic inflammation often manifests in aches, pains, and skin issues.

- **Improved digestion and gut comfort:** Gas, bloating, and irregular bathroom trips should be greatly improved by the end of the protocol. If you used to feel like a balloon after every meal, or lived on anti-diarrhea medication due to an uneasy gut, a restored microbiome and barrier can be life-changing. It's the difference between constantly thinking about your gut versus your gut functioning quietly in the background like it's supposed to.

- **More energy and brighter mood:** Many people report better focus and improved mood as their gut health improves. You may wake up feeling more refreshed and notice fewer of those brain-fog moments. Steadier blood sugar and less immune stress means a calmer, clearer mind.

The outcome we're aiming for is a holistic upgrade to your well-being. You're working toward a healthier weight and a metabolism that's more flexible and resilient. Instead of riding the hunger-energy roller coaster, you're cruising smoothly. Best of all, these wins build on each other: As you feel better, you'll be motivated to keep the healthy habits going. Let's wrap up by comparing this gut-centric approach with the medication route.

Comparison with GLP-1 Drugs—Biohack Your Own GLP-1 Versus Injecting It

Remember our discussion of Ozempic and Wegovy earlier in this book? These medications mimic the GLP-1 hormone to suppress appetite and improve insulin release, essentially doing pharmacologically what our protocol achieves naturally. Let's compare the two approaches.

Similarities

Both can reduce hunger, help you eat less, and improve blood sugar control. People taking GLP-1 shots lose weight for the same fundamental reasons someone on our gut protocol would—they're eating less and their metabolism is working better. Both approaches can lead to lower inflammation and better metabolic health markers. If you use GLP-1 drugs or other prescription meds, talk with your health-care provider before you change doses, stop a drug, or add this protocol. Your plan should fit your medical history and current prescriptions.

Differences

The obvious difference is how we get there. The drug is like an on-switch for GLP-1 receptors—you inject it and force those pathways open. Our protocol, on the other hand, coaxes your body to produce more GLP-1 and other satiety signals on its own, by feeding your gut the right inputs. This means:

- **Fewer side effects:** GLP-1 meds commonly cause nausea, vomiting, diarrhea, or constipation. Some people feel crummy on them all the time. They can also slow stomach emptying to the point that acid reflux or other issues develop. Our gut-focused approach might cause a few transient side effects, but nothing like the medication's GI upheaval. In fact, our aim is to reduce gut discomfort overall.

- **Safety profile:** The drugs are still being studied for long-term safety. There have been rare cases of things such as pancreatitis and gallbladder issues with GLP-1 agonists. Meanwhile, our protocol—improving diet and adding probiotics—is generally very safe and has side benefits, such as better nutrient intake and immune support.

- **Holistic benefits:** Our protocol can improve a broad spectrum of health markers. The injections, while helpful for weight, may not address those other areas.

- **Effort and habits:** Let's be real: It's easier to take a shot once a week than to change your eating habits. The drug doesn't ask you to alter what you eat—at least not initially. Our program does require effort and consistency. You have to plan meals, avoid certain foods, and remember to take supplements (the Mercola Health Coach app will help with these). However, putting in this effort means you're building sustainable habits. Stopping a GLP-1 injection often brings appetite roaring back. Weight can rebound unless you've made lifestyle changes, too. In contrast, the progress you make with a lifestyle approach tends to be more lasting because you've changed your body's baseline and your behaviors.

- **Cost:** GLP-1 drugs are expensive. Without insurance, they can cost more than $1,000 per month. Even with coverage, many people struggle to get them approved unless they have diabetes. Our program costs a fraction of that price. (Plus, you'll save money in the long run by avoiding ultra-processed foods and takeout.)

You can always talk with your health-care provider about combining approaches. Even if you do decide to take a medication, the gut work will amplify your results. I'm a fan of mastering my own biology rather than depending on a prescription for life—and I suspect you are too, since you've read this far!

You've got the knowledge and the plan. Now it's time to put it into action. Let's close out with a quick victory checklist to celebrate how far you've come and keep you motivated for the road ahead.

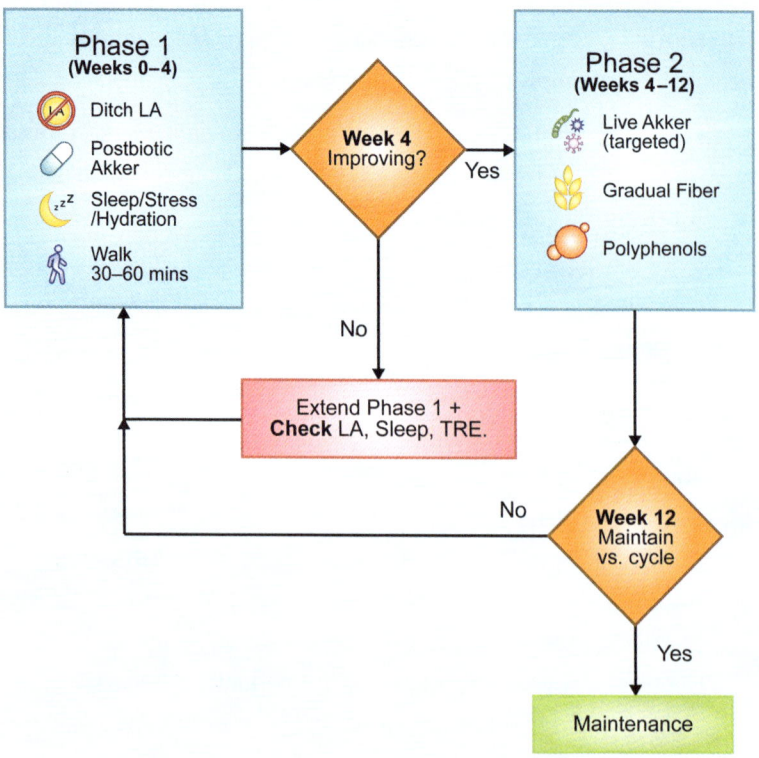

Figure 82. Two-step protocol flowchart showing phase 1 (repair) and phase 2 (reseeding) with feedback loops at weeks 4 and 12.

The Universal Optimization: From Weight-Loss Fix to Many Other Health Wins

Most weight-loss advice focuses on the scale. But the truth is, the same chemistry that drives weight gain also fuels the current epidemics of diabetes, hypertension, arthritis, reflux, depression, fatigue, and even cognitive decline. For decades, we've thrown medications at each of these conditions—statins for cholesterol, proton pump inhibitors (PPIs) for ulcers, selective serotonin reuptake inhibitors (SSRIs) for mood, and metformin for blood sugar. Different pills, different labels, but the same root dysfunction: broken energy production and a gut wall that leaks signals it should be filtering.

The narrative arc here is straightforward: remove the irritant, send the repair signal, then feed the system what it needs to thrive.

> **Step 1:** Cut fragile fats to lower the aldehyde storm and give mitochondria breathing room.
>
> **Step 2:** Bring in pasteurized Akker with its "handshake proteins" (Amuc_1100, P9) to seal the gut wall, thicken mucus, and calm your immune system.
>
> **Step 3:** Make fiber your best friend, but only once the gut wall has healed. Microbes churn fiber into butyrate, oxygen drops, satiety hormones fire naturally, and the whole loop stabilizes.

As a result, that long list of prescriptions starts to look less necessary. Blood sugar steadies, cholesterol normalizes, blood pressure eases, reflux symptoms fade, joints ache less, mood brightens, energy steadies, and infection risk drops. It's not a miracle cure but a return to first principles. The real victory isn't in skipping prescriptions but in no longer needing them at the same dose.

Weight-Loss Conquests: Your Victory Checkpoint

Today's 3-point scorecard:

1. **Consider adding an Akker postbiotic.** A daily capsule sends gut-healing signals that strengthen your barrier and set the stage for metabolic wins.

2. **Do one gentle movement.** Go for a walk, stretch, or try light yoga to support gut motility and calm stress.

3. **Prioritize one lifestyle win.** Decide on a bedtime (and stick to it!) or carve out at least ten minutes or more to wind down before bed. Examples include taking a hot bath or turning down the light and reading a few pages from a good book.

CONCLUSION
From Quick Fixes to Lasting Resilience

Over these chapters, we have met the quiet genius of your microbes. We've met *Akkermansia muciniphila,* especially, the mucus gardener whose presence predicts leaner bodies and less inflammation.

We've explored Gut Gems—those humble SCFAs—such as butyrate—that fuel colon cells, tighten the gut barrier, and encourage your gut to release GLP-1 and PYY, the very satiety hormones billion-dollar drugs mimic.

We've seen how fragile fats, particularly seed oils loaded with LA, corrode this system from the inside out. Their oxidized fragments disrupt colonocyte energy production, leave excess oxygen in the colon, and thin protective mucus in the gut lining.

At the same time, the lack of fiber in modern diets has starved beneficial microbes, weakening the very feedback loops that sustain appetite control and metabolic calm. And we've looked at one of the most counterintuitive findings of all: Sometimes dead bacteria work better than live ones. Pasteurized Akker, stripped of its ability to reproduce, still delivers its proteins and vesicles as potent signals—calming inflammation, boosting insulin sensitivity, and enhancing GLP-1 secretion. Postbiotics, stable and safe, offer a way forward when probiotics and fiber falter.

Taken together, these discoveries point to a new paradigm: Weight loss isn't just about calories in and calories out. It's about repairing the gut's inner ecosystem so that hunger signals, hormone release, and metabolic balance fall back into alignment. When your L cells release GLP-1 and PYY naturally, you eat less without feeling deprived, your blood sugar steadies, and your pancreas doesn't burn out.

Yes, weight loss is a goal. But the gut revolution is about more than inches around the waist. It's about energy, immunity, mood, and long-term resilience. When your colonocytes burn butyrate efficiently, they vacuum up oxygen and preserve the anaerobic environment your best microbes require. When your mucus barrier is thick and intact, toxins such as LPS can't leak into your bloodstream to fuel chronic inflammation.

These are not cosmetic shifts. They are systemic recalibrations that reduce the risk of diabetes, heart disease, fatty liver, autoimmune flares, even certain cancers. In a health-care system straining under the weight of chronic disease, gut repair isn't just personal wellness—it's public health.

It is tempting to believe in shortcuts. The mind loves immediacy—like a fast scale drop or a smaller dress size—and GLP-1 injections fit neatly into that temptation. But while a silenced hunger cue is useful for a season, a repaired gut that generates those signals on its own is useful for a lifetime.

That is why the greatest shift is of the mind. Instead of seeing the gut as a passive food chute, we must treat it as a living organ system responsive to care and neglect. We must think in terms of ecology: balance, diversity, and resilience.

This perspective dissolves the old blame game of willpower and calories. Struggling with weight is not a failing of grit. It is often a symptom of a disrupted inner ecosystem. By repairing that ecosystem, you no longer need to fight yourself. Instead you can focus on restoring the conditions for health. Only a century ago, Élie Metchnikoff—the scientist who discovered phagocytosis—speculated that fermented milk could extend human life by cultivating better microbes. His tools were crude, his conclusions incomplete, but his intuition was right: Longevity flows from the gut.

Today—with genetic sequencing, controlled trials, and biochemical insight—we can finally see what he glimpsed. The gut is not a sideshow in health; it is the main stage. And weight loss, once thought of as a simple math equation, is in reality a negotiation between food, microbes, hormones, and barrier integrity.

The drugs of today have sparked attention, but the future belongs to a holistic approach—one where the gut is treated as a metabolic organ, and not merely a waste chute. If you take nothing else from this book, take this: Your gut is not broken beyond repair. Even decades of fragile fats, fiber neglect, and chronic inflammation can be reversed. Microbes are resilient. Barriers can be rebuilt. Satiety signals can be rekindled.

This is not a call to perfection. It's not a call to eat kale at every meal or swear off fries forever. It is a call for small, consistent choices—swapping oils, adding foods with color, walking after dinner—that ripple inward to change the microbial ecosystem that runs your metabolism. Over weeks, months, and years, these choices repair the gut.

The gut is your oldest ally. Now it is your future.

References: Your Direct Line to the Science (Professional Section)

This book rests on a solid scientific foundation, with many references. If you're a clinician, researcher, or just someone who loves to get into the weeds, this "professional" section is for you. Every claim is traceable, and you can dig deeper into the primary research whenever curiosity strikes.

My goal is to give you more than information: I want to equip you with the tools to think critically, test ideas, and explore the evolving science of health firsthand. That is why you'll find links to the original papers throughout.

Keep in mind, though, that science never stands still. What we know today is the best picture available—but tomorrow's research may refine or even rewrite parts of the story. This book is a guide, not the final word, and these references are your gateway to staying in the conversation.

Chapter 1: Weight-Loss Breakthroughs: From Miracle Meds to Microbiome Magic
1. Liu, Qiyuan Keith. "Mechanisms of Action and Therapeutic Applications of GLP-1 and Dual GIP/GLP-1 Receptor Agonists." *Frontiers in Endocrinology* 15 (2024): 1431292.
2. Drucker, Daniel J. "Mechanisms of Action and Therapeutic Application of Glucagon-Like Peptide-1." *Cell Metabolism* 27, no. 4 (2018): 740–56.

3. Maselli, Daniel B., and Michael Camilleri. "Effects of GLP-1 and Its Analogs on Gastric Physiology in Diabetes Mellitus and Obesity." *Advances in Experimental Medicine and Biology* 1307 (2021).

4. Hall, Kevin D. "Physiology of the Weight-Loss Plateau in Response to Diet Restriction, GLP-1 Receptor Agonism, and Bariatric Surgery." *Obesity* 32, no. 6 (2024).

5. Wilding, John P. H., Rachel L. Batterham, Melanie Davies et al. "Weight Regain and Cardiometabolic Effects after Withdrawal of Semaglutide: The STEP 1 Trial Extension." *Diabetes, Obesity and Metabolism* 24, no. 8 (2022): 1553–64.

6. Ushakumari, Deepu S., and Robert N. Sladen. "ASA Consensus-Based Guidance on Preoperative Management of Patients on Glucagon-Like Peptide-1 Receptor Agonists." *Anesthesiology* 140, no. 2 (2024): 346–8.

7. He, Liyun, Jialu Wang, Fan Ping et al. "Association of Glucagon-Like Peptide-1 Receptor Agonist Use With Risk of Gallbladder and Biliary Diseases: A Systematic Review and Meta-Analysis of Randomized Clinical Trials." *JAMA Internal Medicine* 182, no. 5 (2022): 513–19.

8. Tobaiqy, Mohammed, and Hadeel Elkout. "Psychiatric Adverse Events Associated with Semaglutide, Liraglutide and Tirzepatide: A Pharmacovigilance Analysis of Individual Case Safety Reports Submitted to the EudraVigilance Database." *International Journal of Clinical Pharmacy* 46, no. 2 (2024): 488–95.

9. Aronne, Louis J., Naveed Sattar, Deborah B. Horn et al. "Continued Treatment with Tirzepatide for Maintenance of Weight Reduction in Adults with Obesity: The SURMOUNT-4 Randomized Clinical Trial." *JAMA* 331, no. 1 (2024): 38–48.

10. Park, J. S., Kwang S. Kim, and Hee J. Choi. "Glucagon-Like Peptide-1 and Hypothalamic Regulation of Satiation: Cognitive and Neural Insights from Human and Animal Studies." *Diabetes & Metabolism Journal* 49, no. 3 (2025): 333–47.

11. Derrien, Muriel, Elaine E. Vaughan, Caroline M. Plugge, and Willem M. de Vos. "*Akkermansia muciniphila* gen. nov., sp. nov., a Human Intestinal Mucin-Degrading Bacterium." *International Journal of Systematic Evolutionary Microbiology* 54, pt. 5 (2004): 1469–76.

12. Liu, Meng-Jie, Jing-Yu Yang, Zhen-Hua Yan et al. "Recent Findings in *Akkermansia muciniphila*-Regulated Metabolism and Its

Role in Intestinal Diseases." *Clinical Nutrition* 41, no. 10 (2022): 2333–44.

13. Gustafsson, Jenny K., and Malin E. V. Johansson. "The Role of Goblet Cells and Mucus in Intestinal Homeostasis." *Nature Reviews Gastroenterol & Hepatology* 19, no.12 (2022): 785–803.

14. Blaak, Ellen E., E. E. Canfora, S. Theis et al. "Short Chain Fatty Acids in Human Gut and Metabolic Health." *Beneficial Microbes* 11, no. 5 (2020): 411–55.

15. Du, Yuhang, Changhao He, Yongcheng An et al. "The Role of Short-Chain Fatty Acids in Inflammation and Body Health." *International Journal of Molecular Sciences* 25, no. 13 (2024): 7379, https://www.ncbi.nlm.nih.gov/pmc/articles/PMC11242198/.

16. Everard, Amandine, Clara Belzer, Lucie Geurts et al. "Cross-Talk Between *Akkermansia muciniphila* and Intestinal Epithelium Controls Diet-Induced Obesity." *Proceedings of the National Academy of Sciences of the United States of America* 110, no. 22 (2013): 9066–71.

17. Yan, Juan, Lili Sheng, and Houkai Li. "*Akkermansia muciniphila*: Is It the Holy Grail for Ameliorating Metabolic Diseases?" *Gut Microbes* 13, no. 1 (2021): 1984104.

18. Zhou, Qi, Guofang Pang, Zhirong Zhang et al. "Association Between Gut *Akkermansia* and Metabolic Syndrome Is Dose-Dependent and Affected by Microbial Interactions: A Cross-Sectional Study." *Diabetes, Metabolic Syndrome and Obesity: Targets and Therapy* 14 (May 2021): 2177–88.

19. Depommier, Clara, Amandine Everard, Celine Druart et al. "Supplementation with *Akkermansia muciniphila* in Overweight and Obese Human Volunteers: A Proof-of-Concept Exploratory Study." *Nature Medicine* 25, no. 7 (2019): 1096–103.

20. Cani, Patrice D., Clara Depommier, Muriel Derrien et al. "*Akkermansia muciniphila*: Paradigm for Next-Generation Beneficial Microorganisms." *Nature Reviews Gastroenterology & Hepatology* 19, no. 10 (2022): 625–37.

21. Mruk-Mazurkiewicz, Honorata, Monika Kulaszynska, Wiktoria Czarnecka et al. "Insights into the Mechanisms of Action of *Akkermansia muciniphila* in the Treatment of Non-Communicable Diseases," *Nutrients* 16, no. 11 (2024): 1695.

22. Turck, Dominique, Torsten Bohn, Jacqueline Castenmiller et al. "Safety of Pasteurised *Akkermansia muciniphila* as a Novel Food Pursuant to Regulation (EU) 2015/2283." *EFSA Journal* 19, no. 9 (2021): e06780.

23. Chiantera, Vito, Antonio Simone Lagana, Sabrina Basciani, Maurizio Nordio, and Mariano Bizzarri. "Critical Perspective on the Supplementation of *Akkermansia muciniphila*: Benefits and Harms." *Life* 13, no. 6 (2023): 1247.

24. Van Buiten, Charlene B., Valerie A. Seitz, Jessica L. Metcalf, and Ilya Raskin. "Dietary Polyphenols Support *Akkermansia muciniphila* Growth via Mediation of the Gastrointestinal Redox Environment." *Antioxidants* 13, no. 3 (2024): 304.

25. Tingler, Anna M., and Melinda A. Engevik. "Breaking Down Barriers: Is Intestinal Mucus Degradation by *Akkermansia muciniphila* Beneficial or Harmful?" *Infection and Immunity* (2025): e0050324.

26. Torres, Belen, Maria C. Sanchez, Leire Virto et al. "Use of Probiotics in Preventing and Treating Excess Weight and Obesity: A Systematic Review." *Obesity Science & Practice* 10, no. 3 (2024): e759.

27. Sender, Ron, Shai Fuchs, and Ron Milo. "Revised Estimates for the Number of Human and Bacteria Cells in the Body." *PLoS Biology* 14, no. 8 (2016): e1002533.

28. Andrade, Jose Carlos, Diana Almeida, Melany Domingos et al. "Commensal Obligate Anaerobic Bacteria and Health: Production, Storage, and Delivery Strategies." *Frontiers in Bioengineering and Biotechnology* 8 (2020): 550.

29. Sardelli, Lorenzo, Simone Petrottoni, Marta Tunesi et al. "Technological Tools and Strategies for Culturing Human Gut Microbiota in Engineered in Vitro Models." *Biotechnology and Bioengineering* 118, no. 8 (2021): 2886–905.

30. Walaas, Gunner Andreas, Shreya Gopalakrishnan, Ingunn Bakke et al. "Physiological Hypoxia Improves Growth and Functional Differentiation of Human Intestinal Epithelial Organoids." *Frontiers in Immunology* 14 (2023): 1095812.

31. Patel, Dhruvesh, Jenna Evanchuk, Ren Wang et al. "Regulation of Immune Function in Healthy Adults: One-Stop Guide on the

Role of Dietary Fatty Acids, Gut Microbiota-Derived Short Chain Fatty Acids, and Select Micronutrients in Combination with Physical Activity." *Applied Physiology, Nutrition, and Metabolism* 48, no. 8 (2023): 554–68.

32. Poto, Remo, William Fusco, Emanuele Rinninella et al. "The Role of Gut Microbiota and Leaky Gut in the Pathogenesis of Food Allergy." *Nutrients* 16, no. 1 (2023): 92.

33. Colella, Marica, Ioannis Alexandros Charitos, Andrea Ballini et al. "Microbiota Revolution: How Gut Microbes Regulate Our Lives." *World Journal of Gastroenterology* 29, no. 28 (2023): 4368–83.

34. Liu, Xiao-feng, Jia-hao Shao, Yi-Tao Liao et al. "Regulation of Short-Chain Fatty Acids in the Immune System." *Frontiers in Immunology* 14 (2023): 1186892.

35. Baldelli, Valerio, Franco Scaldaferri, Lorenza Putignani, and Federica Del Chierico. "The Role of Enterobacteriaceae in Gut Microbiota Dysbiosis in Inflammatory Bowel Diseases." *Microorganisms* 9, no. 4 (2021): 697.

36. Fagundes, Raphael, Saskia C. Belt, Barbara M. Bakker et al. "Beyond Butyrate: Microbial Fiber Metabolism Supporting Colonic Epithelial Homeostasis." *Trends in Microbiology* 32, no. 2 (2024): 178–89.

37. Salvi, Pooja S. and Robert A. Cowles. "Butyrate and the Intestinal Epithelium: Modulation of Proliferation and Inflammation in Homeostasis and Disease." *Cells* 10, no. 7 (2021): 1775.

38. Fu, Jiongxing, Yan Zheng, Ying Gao, and Wanghong Xu. "Dietary Fiber Intake and Gut Microbiota in Human Health." *Microorganisms* 10, no. 12 (2022): 2507.

39. Wan, Xuchun, Qianqian Yang, Xiangfeng Wang, Yun Bai, and Zhi Liu. "Isolation and Cultivation of Human Gut Microorganisms: A Review." *Microorganisms* 11, no. 4 (2023): 1080.

40. Meyers, Guilherme Ramos, Hanen Samouda, and Torsten Bohn. "Short Chain Fatty Acid Metabolism in Relation to Gut Microbiota and Genetic Variability." *Nutrients* 14, no. 24 (2022): 5361.

41. Singhal, Rashi, and Yatrik M. Shah. "Oxygen Battle in the Gut: Hypoxia and Hypoxia-Inducible Factors in Metabolic and Inflammatory Responses in the Intestine." *Journal of Biological Chemistry* 295, no. 30 (2020): 10493–505.

42. Pohl, Keith, Prebashan Moodley, and Aashwin Dhanda. "The Effect of Increasing Intestinal Short-Chain Fatty Acid Concentration on Gut Permeability and Liver Injury in the Context of Liver Disease: A Systematic Review." *Journal of Gastroenterology and Hepatology* 37, no. 8 (2022): 1498–506.

43. Liu, Pinyi, Yangbing Wang, Ge Yang et al. "The Role of Short-Chain Fatty Acids in Intestinal Barrier Function, Inflammation, Oxidative Stress, and Colonic Carcinogenesis." *Pharmacological Research* 165 (2021): 105420.

44. Jung, Tae-Hwan, Kyoung-Sik Han, Jeong-Hyeon Park, and Hyo-Jeong Hwang. "Butyrate Modulates Mucin Secretion and Bacterial Adherence in LoVo Cells via MAPK Signaling." *PloS One* 17, no. 7 (2022): e0269872.

45. Pham, Nhan H. T., Mugdha V. Joglekar, Wilson K. M. Wong et al. "Short-Chain Fatty Acids and Insulin Sensitivity: A Systematic Review and Meta-Analysis." *Nutrition Reviews* 82, no. 2 (2024): 193–209.

46. Donohoe, Dallas R., Nikhil Garge et al. "The Microbiome and Butyrate Regulate Energy Metabolism and Autophagy in the Mammalian Colon." *Cell Metabolism* 13, no. 5 (2011): 517–26.

47. Winter, Sebastian E., and Andreas J. Bäumler. "Gut Dysbiosis: Ecological Causes and Causative Effects on Human Disease." *Proceedings of the National Academy of Sciences of the United States of America* 120, no. 50 (2023): e2316579120.

48. Ghosh Sweta, Caleb Samuel Whitley, Bodduluri Haribabu, and Venkatakrishna Rao Jala. "Regulation of Intestinal Barrier Function by Microbial Metabolites." *Cellular and Molecular Gastroenterology and Hepatology* 11, no. 5 (2021): 1463–82.

49. Siddiqui, Mohamed Tausif, and Gail A. M. Cresci. "The Immunomodulatory Functions of Butyrate." *Journal of Inflammation Research* 14 (2021): 6025–41.

50. Vinelli, Valentina, Paola Biscotti, Daniela Martini et al. "Effects of Dietary Fibers on Short-Chain Fatty Acids and Gut Microbiota Composition in Healthy Adults: A Systematic Review." *Nutrients* 14, no. 13 (2022): 2559.

51. Lee, Joyce H., Miranda Duster, Timothy Roberts, and Orrin Devinsky. "United States Dietary Trends Since 1800: Lack of Association Between Saturated Fatty Acid Consumption and Non-Communicable Diseases." *Frontiers in Nutrition* 8 (2022): 748847.

52. Deol, Poonamjot, Paul Ruegger, Geoffrey D. Logan et al. "Diet High in Linoleic Acid Dysregulates the Intestinal Endocannabinoid System and Increases Susceptibility to Colitis in Mice." *Gut Microbes* 15, no. 1 (2023): 2229945.

53. Mititelu, Magdalena, Dumitru Lupuliassa, Sorinel Marius Neacsu et al. "Polyunsaturated Fatty Acids and Human Health: A Key to Modern Nutritional Balance in Association with Polyphenolic Compounds from Food Sources." *Foods* 14, no. 1 (2024): 46.

54. Zhuang, Yuan, Jun Dong, Xiaomei He et al. "Impact of Heating Temperature and Fatty Acid Type on the Formation of Lipid Oxidation Products During Thermal Processing." *Frontiers in Nutrition* 9 (2022): 913297.

55. Li, Yanling, Tingting Zhao, Jiaxin Li et al. "Oxidative Stress and 4-Hydroxy-2-Nonenal (4-HNE): Implications in the Pathogenesis and Treatment of Aging-Related Diseases." *Journal of Immunology Research* (2022): 2233906.

56. Muro, Peter, Li Zhang, Shuxuan Li et al. "The Emerging Role of Oxidative Stress in Inflammatory Bowel Disease." *Frontiers in Endocrinology* 15 (2024): 1390351.

57. Guimaraes, Kisian Costa, Catarina Mendes Silva, Carolina de Oliveira Cruz Latorraca et al. "Is Self-Reported Short Sleep Duration Associated with Obesity? A Systematic Review and Meta-Analysis of Cohort Studies." *Nutrition Reviews* 80, no. 5 (2022): 983–1000.

58. Abrante-Pascual, Susana, Barbara Nieva-Echevarría, and Encarnación Goicoochea-Oses. "Vegetable Oils and Their Use for Frying: A Review of Their Compositional Differences and Degradation." *Foods* 13, no. 24 (2024): 4186.

59. Seino, Yusuke, and Yuji Yamazaki. "Roles of Glucose-Dependent Insulinotropic Polypeptide in Diet-Induced Obesity." *Journal of Diabetes Investigation* 13, no. 7 (2022): 1122–28.

60. Santos-Hernández, Marta, Frank Reimann, and Fiona M. Gribble. "Cellular Mechanisms of Incretin Hormone Secretion." *Journal of Molecular Endocrinology* 72, no. 4 (2024): e230112.

61. Wolever, Thomas M. S., Susan M. Tosh, Susan E. Spruill et al. "Increasing Oat β-glucan Viscosity in a Breakfast Meal Slows Gastric Emptying and Reduces Glycemic and Insulinemic Responses but Has No Effect on Appetite, Food Intake, or Plasma

Ghrelin and PYY Responses in Healthy Humans: A Randomized, Placebo-Controlled, Crossover Trial." *American Journal of Clinical Nutrition* 111, no. 2 (2020): 319–28.

62. Pironi, L., V. Stanghellini, M. Miglioli et al. "Fat-Induced Ileal Brake in Humans: A Dose-Dependent Phenomenon Correlated to the Plasma Levels of Peptide YY." *Gastroenterology* 105, no. 3 (1993): 733–39.

63. Cani, Patrice D., and Claude Knauf. "A Newly Identified Protein from *Akkermansia muciniphila* Stimulates GLP-1 Secretion." *Cell Metabolism* 33, no. 6 (2021): 1073–5.

64. Zeng, Yuan, Yifan Wu, Qian Zhang, and Xinhua Xiao. "Crosstalk Between Glucagon-Like Peptide 1 and Gut Microbiota in Metabolic Diseases." *MBio* 15, no. 1 (2024): e0203223.

65. Rodríguez-Daza, Maria Carolina, and Willem M. de Vos. "Polyphenols as Drivers of a Homeostatic Gut Microecology and Immuno-Metabolic Traits of *Akkermansia muciniphila*: From Mouse to Man." *International Journal of Molecular Sciences* 24, no 1 (2022): 45.

66. Vinderola, Gabriel, Mary Ellen Sanders, Marla Cunningham, and Colin Hill. "Frequently Asked Questions About the ISAPP Postbiotic Definition." *Frontiers in Microbiology* 14 (2024): 1324565.

67. Salminen, Seppo, Maria Carmen Collado, Akihito Endo et al. "The International Scientific Association of Probiotics and Prebiotics (ISAPP) Consensus Statement on the Definition and Scope of Postbiotics." *Nature Reviews Gastroenterology & Hepatology* 18, no. 9 (2021): 649–67.

68. Hijová, Emilia. "Postbiotics as Metabolites and Their Biotherapeutic Potential." *International Journal of Molecular Sciences* 25, no. 10 (2024): 5441.

69. Jastrząb, Rafal, Damian Graczyk, and Pawel Siedlecki. "Molecular and Cellular Mechanisms Influenced by Postbiotics." *International Journal of Molecular Sciences* 22, no. 24 (2021): 13475.

70. He, Kairu, Feiyu An, Henan Zhang et al. "*Akkermansia muciniphila*: A Potential Target for the Prevention of Diabetes." *Foods* 14, no. 1 (2024): 23.

71. Plovier, Hubert, Amandine Everard, Celine Druart et al. "A Purified Membrane Protein from *Akkermansia muciniphila* or the Pasteurized Bacterium Improves Metabolism in Obese and Diabetic Mice." *Nature Medicine* 23, no. 1 (2017): 107–13.

72. Liang, Bing, and Dongming Xing. "The Current and Future Perspectives of Postbiotics. Probiotics Antimicrobial Proteins." *Probiotics and Antimicrobial Proteins* (2023): 1–18.

73. Wang, Shi, Weibing Wu, Zhengwei Chen, Chaobo Xu, Kai Zhang, and Xiaoya Xu. "The Effect of Probiotics on Weight Management in Patients with Severe Obesity Undergoing Metabolic and Bariatric Surgery: A Systematic Review and Meta-Analysis." *Annals of Medicine* 57, no. 1 (2025): 2551284. doi:10.1080/07853890.2025.2551284.

74. Magryś, Agnieszka, and Mateusz Pawlik. "Postbiotic Fractions of Probiotics *Lactobacillus plantarum* 299v and *Lactobacillus rhamnosus* GG Show Immune-Modulating Effects." *Cells* 12, no. 21 (2023): 2538.

75. Kato, Kumiko, Satoshi Arai, Soichiro Sato et al. "Effects of Heat-Killed *Lacticaseibacillus paracasei* MCC1849 on Immune Parameters in Healthy Adults—a Randomized, Double-Blind, Placebo-Controlled, Parallel-Group Study." *Nutrients* 16, no. 2 (2024): 216.

76. Nobutani, K., D. Sawada, S. Fujiwara et al. "The Effects of Administration of the *Lactobacillus gasseri* Strain CP2305 on Quality of Life, Clinical Symptoms and Changes in Gene Expression in Patients with Irritable Bowel Syndrome." *Journal of Applied Microbiology* 122, no. 1 (2017): 212–24.

77. Wei, Li, Botao Wang, Junying Bai et al. "Postbiotics Are a Candidate for New Functional Foods." *Food Chemistry: X* 23 (2024): 101650.

78. Yang, Xinyuan, Chong Wang, Qiao Wang et al. "Armored Probiotics for Oral Delivery." *Smart Medicine* 2, no. 4 (2023): e20230019.

79. Treven, Primoz, Diana Paveljsek, Bojana Bogovic Matijasic, and Petra Mohar Lorbeg. "The Effect of Food Matrix Taken with Probiotics on the Survival of Commercial Probiotics in Simulation of Gastrointestinal Digestion." *Foods* 13, no. 19 (2024): 3135.

80. Chai, Li-Na, Hua Wu, Xue-Jiao Wang, Li-Juan He, and Chun-Feng Guo. "The Mechanism of Antimicrobial Activity of Conjugated Bile Acids Against Lactic Acid Bacilli." *Microorganisms* 11, no. 7 (2023): 1823.

81. Lu, Zheng, and James A. Imlay. "When Anaerobes Encounter Oxygen: Mechanisms of Oxygen Toxicity, Tolerance and Defence." *Nature Reviews Microbiology* 19, no. 12 (2021): 774–85.

82. Gvozdeva, Yana, and Radiana Staynova. "pH-Dependent Drug Delivery Systems for Ulcerative Colitis Treatment." *Pharmaceutics* 17, no. 2 (2025): 226.

83. Wang, Xiaochen, Shukun Gao, Shuaiting Yun et al. "Microencapsulating Alginate-Based Polymers for Probiotics Delivery Systems and Their Application." *Pharmaceuticals* 15, no. 5 (2022): 644.

84. Govaert, Marlies, Chloe Rotsaert, Chelsea Vannieuwenhuyse et al. "Survival of Probiotic Bacterial Cells in the Upper Gastrointestinal Tract and the Effect of the Surviving Population on the Colonic Microbial Community Activity and Composition." *Nutrients* 16, no. 16 (2024): 2791.

85. Mortensen, Alicja, Fernando Aquilar, Riccardo Crebelli et al. "Re-evaluation of Konjac Gum (E 425 i) and Konjac Glucomannan (E 425 ii) as Food Additives." *EFSA Journal* 15, no. 6 (2017): e04864.

86. Agriopoulou, Sofia, Maria Tarapoulouzi, Theodoros Varzakas, and Seid Mahdi Jafari. "Application of Encapsulation Strategies for Probiotics: From Individual Loading to Co-Encapsulation." *Microorganisms* 11, no. 12 (2023): 2896.

87. Malcomson, Fiona C., Panayiotis Louca, Andrew Nelson et al. "Effects of Non-Digestible Carbohydrates on Gut Microbiota and Microbial Metabolites: A Randomised, Controlled Dietary Intervention in Healthy Individuals." *British Journal of Nutrition* 132, no. 11 (2024): 1433–45.

88. Guan, Zhi-Wei, En-Ze Yu, and Qiang Feng. "Soluble Dietary Fiber, One of the Most Important Nutrients for the Gut Microbiota." *Molecules* 26, no. 22 (2021): 6802.

89. Van der Schoot, Alice, Candice Drysdale, Kevin Whelan, and Eirini Dimidi. "The Effect of Fiber Supplementation on Chronic Constipation in Adults: An Updated Systematic Review and Meta-Analysis of Randomized Controlled Trials." *American Journal of Clinical Nutrition,* 116, no. 4 (2022): 953–69.

90. Wang, Zhanggui, Shuli Wang, Qinhong Xu et al. "Synthesis and Functions of Resistant Starch." *Advances in Nutrition* 14, no. 5 (2023): 1131–44.

91. Chen, Zhao, Ning Liang, Haili Zhang et al. "Resistant Starch and the Gut Microbiome: Exploring Beneficial Interactions and Dietary Impacts." *Food Chemistry: X* (2024): 101118.

92. Mysonhimer, Annemarie R., and Hannah D. Holscher. "Gastrointestinal Effects and Tolerance of Nondigestible Carbohydrate Consumption." *Advances in Nutrition* 13, no. 6 (2022): 2237–76.

93. Di Vincenzo, Federica, Angelo Del Gaudio, Valentina Petito, Loris Riccardo Lopetuso, and Franco Scaldaferri. "Gut Microbiota, Intestinal Permeability, and Systemic Inflammation: A Narrative Review." *Internal Emergency Medicine* 19, no. 2 (2024): 275–93.

94. Wang, Xiaofei, Yue Qi, and Hao Zheng. "Dietary Polyphenol, Gut Microbiota, and Health Benefits." *Antioxidants* 11, no. 6 (2022): 1212.

95. Scianò, Fabio, Bianca Laura Bernadoni, Ilaria D'Agostino et al. "Toxic Aldehydes in Cooking Vegetable Oils: Generation, Toxicity and Disposal Methods." *Food Chemistry: X* 29 (2025): 102744.

96. Daniel, Noemie, Andrew T. Gewirtz, and Benoit Chassaing. "*Akkermansia muciniphila* Counteracts the Deleterious Effects of Dietary Emulsifiers on Microbiota and Host Metabolism." *Gut* 72, no. 5 (2023): 906–17.

97. Ramar, Kannan, Raman K. Malhotra, Kelly A Carden et al. "Sleep Is Essential to Health: An American Academy of Sleep Medicine Position Statement." *Journal of Clinical Sleep Medicine* 17, no. 10 (2021): 2115–9.

98. La Torre, Danique, Lukas Van Oudenhove, Tim Vanuytsel, and Kristin Verbeke. "Psychosocial Stress-Induced Intestinal Permeability in Healthy Humans: What Is the Evidence?" *Neurobiology of Stress* 27 (2023): 100579.

99. Al-Beltagi, Mohammed, Nermin Kamal Saeed, Adel Salah Bediwy et al. "Exploring the Gut-Exercise Link: A Systematic Review of Gastrointestinal Disorders in Physical Activity." *World Journal of Gastroenterology* 31, no. 22 (2025): 106835.

100. Sato, Kensuke, Mariko Hara-Chikuma, Masato Yasui, Joe Inoue, and Yun-Gi Kim. "Sufficient Water Intake Maintains the Gut Microbiota and Immune Homeostasis and Promotes Pathogen Elimination." *iScience* 27, no. 6 (2024): 109903.

101. Jan, Tawseefa, Rajeshwari Negi, Babita Sharma et al. "Next Generation Probiotics for Human Health: An Emerging Perspective." *Heliyon* 10, no. 16 (2024): e35980.

102. Daneshgaran, Giulia, Orr Shauly, Daniel J. Gould. "'Ozempic Face' in Plastic Surgery: A Systematic Review of the Literature

on GLP-1 Receptor Agonist-Mediated Weight Loss and Analysis of Public Perceptions." *Aesthetic Surgery Journal Open Forum* 7 (2025): ojaf056.

Chapter 2: GLP-1 Drugs: A Consumer-Friendly Blueprint

1. Nauck, Michael A., Daniel R. Quest, Jakob Wefers, and Juris J. Meier. "GLP-1 Receptor Agonists in the Treatment of Type 2 Diabetes—State-of-the-Art." *Molecular Metabolism* 46 (2020): 101102.

2. Sodum, Nalini, Orvokki Mattila, Ravikant Sharma et al. "Nutrient Combinations Sensed by L-Cell Receptors Potentiate GLP-1 Secretion." *International Journal of Molecular Sciences* 25, no. 2 (2024): 1087.

3. Wilding, John P. H., Rachel L. Batterham, Salvatore Calanna et al. "Once-Weekly Semaglutide in Adults with Overweight or Obesity." *New England Journal of Medicine* 384, no. 11 (2021): 989–1002.

4. Amaro, Anastassia, Danny Sugimoto, and Sean Wharton. "Efficacy and Safety of Semaglutide for Weight Management: Evidence from the STEP Program." *Postgraduate Medicine* 134, suppl. 1 (2022): 5–17.

5. Fornes, Abby, Jamie Huff, Roer Iain Pritchard, and Miranda Godfrey. "Once-Weekly Semaglutide for Weight Management: A Clinical Review." *Journal of Pharmacy Technology* 38, no. 4 (2022): 239–46, https://www.ncbi.nlm.nih.gov/pmc/articles/PMC 9272494/.

6. Wilding, John P. H., Rachel L. Batterham, Melanie Davies et al. "Weight Regain and Cardiometabolic Effects After Withdrawal of Semaglutide: The STEP 1 Trial Extension." *Diabetes, Obesity and Metabolism* 24, no. 8 (2022): 1553–64.

7. Jalleh, Ryan J., Mark P. Plummer, Chinmay S. Marathe et al. "Clinical Consequences of Delayed Gastric Emptying with GLP-1 Receptor Agonists and Tirzepatide." *Journal of Clinical Endocrinology and Metabolism* 110, no. 1 (2024): 1–15.

8. Kim, Kyu Sik, Joon Seok Park, Eunsang Hwang et al. "GLP-1 Increases Preingestive Satiation via Hypothalamic Circuits in Mice and Humans." *Science* 385, no. 6707 (2024): 438–46.

9. Chiang, Cho-Hung, Aunchalee Jaroenlapnopparat, Sena Cakir Colak et al. "Glucagon-Like Peptide-1 Receptor Agonists

and Gastrointestinal Adverse Events: A Systematic Review and Meta-Analysis." *Gastroenterology* (June 9, 2025): S0016-5085(25)00845-5.

10. Ismaiel, Abdulrahman, Giuseppe Guido Maria Scarlata, Irina Boitos et al. "Gastrointestinal Adverse Events Associated with GLP-1 RA in Non-Diabetic Patients with Overweight or Obesity: A Systematic Review and Network Meta-Analysis." *International Journal of Obesity* (August 13, 2025).

11. Gariani, Karim, and Alessandro Putzu. "Glucagon-Like Peptide-1 Receptor Agonists in the Perioperative Period: Implications for the Anaesthesiologist." *European Journal of Anaesthesiology* 41, no. 3 (2024): 245–46.

12. Liu, Qiyuan Keith. "Mechanisms of Action and Therapeutic Applications of GLP-1 and Dual GIP/GLP-1 Receptor Agonists." *Frontiers in Endocrinology* 15 (2024): 1431292.

13. Alfaris, Nasreen, Stephanie Waldrop, Veronica Johnson et al. "GLP-1 Single, Dual, and Triple Receptor Agonists for Treating Type 2 Diabetes and Obesity: A Narrative Review." *EClinicalMedicine* 75 (2024): 102782.

14. Jones, Lauren A., and Daniel I. Brierley. "GLP-1 and the Neurobiology of Eating Control: Recent Advances." *Endocrinology* 166, no. 2 (2025): bqae167.

15. DeBenedictis, Julie Nicole, Siren Nymo, Karoline Haagensli Ollestad et al. "Changes in the Homeostatic Appetite System After Weight Loss Reflect a Normalization Toward a Lower Body Weight." *Journal of Clinical Endocrinology and Metabolism* 105, no. 7 (2020): e2538–46.

16. Tzoulis, Ploutarchos, and Stephanie E. Baldeweg. "Semaglutide for Weight Loss: Unanswered Questions." *Frontiers in Endocrinology* 15 (2024): 1382814.

17. Grunvald, Eduardo, Raj Shah, Ruben Hernaez et al. "AGA Clinical Practice Guideline on Pharmacological Interventions for Adults with Obesity." *Gastroenterology* 163, no. 5 (2022): 1198–225.

18. Wharton, Sean, Salvatore Calanna, Melanie Davies et al. "Gastrointestinal Tolerability of Once-Weekly Semaglutide 2.4 mg in Adults with Overweight or Obesity, and the Relationship Between Gastrointestinal Adverse Events and Weight Loss." *Diabetes, Obesity and Metabolism* 24, no. 1 (2022): 94–105.

19. Gorgojo-Martínez, Juan J., Pedro Mezquita-Raya, Juana Carretero-Gomez et al. "Clinical Recommendations to Manage Gastrointestinal Adverse Events in Patients Treated with GLP-1 Receptor Agonists: A Multidisciplinary Expert Consensus." *Journal of Clinical Medicine* 12, no. 1 (2022): 145.

20. Shankar, Aditi, Aditi Sharma, Ariel Vinas, and Robert J. Chilton. "GLP-1 Receptor Agonists and Delayed Gastric Emptying: Implications for Invasive Cardiac Interventions and Surgery." *Cardiovascular Endocrinology and Metabolism* 14, no. 1 (2025): e00321.

21. Mansour, Meghan, Olivia M. Hannawa, Marissa M. Yaldo, Emmanuel M. Nageeb, and Kongkrit Chaiyasate. "The Rise of 'Ozempic Face': Analyzing Trends and Treatment Challenges Associated with Rapid Facial Weight Loss Induced by GLP-1 Agonists." *Journal of Plastic, Reconstructive & Aesthetic Surgery* 96 (2024): 225–27.

22. Camilleri, Michael, Braden Kuo, Linda Nguyen et al. "ACG Clinical Guideline: Gastroparesis." *American Journal of Gastroenterology* 117, no. 8 (2022): 1197–220.

23. Sodhi, Mohit, Ramin Rezaeianzadeh, Abbas Kezouh, and Mahya Etminan. "Risk of Gastrointestinal Adverse Events Associated with Glucagon-Like Peptide-1 Receptor Agonists for Weight Loss." *JAMA* 330, no. 18 (2023): 1795–97.

24. Vilz, Tim O., Burkhard Stoffels, Christian Strassburg, Hans H. Schild, and Jorg C. Kalff. "Ileus in Adults." *Deutsches Ärzteblatt International* 114, nos. 29–30 (2017): 508–18.

25. "FDA Updates Ozempic Label With Warning for Intestinal Blockages." *DiaTribe*, accessed September 15, 2025, https://diatribe.org/diabetes-medications/fda-updates-ozempic-label-warning-intestinal-blockages.

26. Tenner, Scott, Santhi Swaroop Vege, Sunil Sheth et al. "American College of Gastroenterology Guidelines: Management of Acute Pancreatitis." *American Journal of Gastroenterology* 119, no. 3 (2024): 419–37.

27. Espinosa De Ycaza, Anna E., Juan P. Brito, Rozalina C. McCoy, Hui Shao, and Naykky Singh Ospina. "Glucagon-Like Peptide-1 Receptor Agonists and Thyroid Cancer: A Narrative Review." *Thyroid* 34, no. 4 (2024): 403–18.

28. Kelly, Clare A., and Jennifer A. Sipos. "Approach to the Patient with Thyroid Nodules: Considering GLP-1 Receptor Agonists." *Journal of Clinical Endocrinology and Metabolism* 110, no. 6 (2025): e2080–87.

29. Nogueiro, Jorge, Hugo Santos-Sousa, Miguel Ribeiro et al. "Incidence of Symptomatic Gallstones After Bariatric Surgery: The Impact of Expectant Management." *Langenbeck's Archives of Surgery* 408, no. 1 (2023): 160.

30. He, Liyun, Jialu Wang, Na Yang et al. "Association of Glucagon-Like Peptide-1 Receptor Agonist Use with Risk of Gallbladder and Biliary Diseases: A Systematic Review and Meta-Analysis of Randomized Clinical Trials." *JAMA Internal Medicine* 182, no. 5 (2022): 513–19.

31. Natividade, Gabriella R., Bernardo F. Spiazzi, Matheus W. Baumgarten et al. "Ocular Adverse Events with Semaglutide: A Systematic Review and Meta-Analysis." *JAMA Ophthalmology* (August 14, 2025), https://pubmed.ncbi.nlm.nih.gov/40810985/.

32. Hathaway, Jimena T., Madhura P. Shah, David B. Hathaway et al. "Risk of Nonarteritic Anterior Ischemic Optic Neuropathy in Patients Prescribed Semaglutide." *JAMA Ophthalmology* 142, no. 8 (2024): 732–39.

33. Colella-Walsh, Stephanie, and Martin Schrama. "What to Know about the Latest Updates in Ozempic and Wegovy Lawsuits." *JD Supra*, accessed September 15, 2025, https://www.jdsupra.com/legalnews/what-to-know-about-the-latest-updates-1480947/.

34. King, Robert. "Trulicity Lawsuit—September 2025 Update," *King Law*, accessed September 15, 2025, https://www.robertkinglawfirm.com/personal-injury/trulicity-lawsuit/.

35. Salvetat, Maria Letizia, Francesco Pellegrini, Leopoldo Spadea, Carlo Salati, and Marco Zeppieri. "Non-Arteritic Anterior Ischemic Optic Neuropathy (NA-AION): A Comprehensive Overview." *Vision (Basel)* 7, no. 4 (2023): 72.

36. Hsu, Alan Y., Hou-Ting Kuo, Yu-Hsun Wang et al. "Semaglutide and Nonarteritic Anterior Ischemic Optic Neuropathy Risk Among Patients with Diabetes." *JAMA Ophthalmology* 143, no. 5 (2025): 400–407.

37. Lixi, Filippo, Valerio Calabresi, Feyza Cukuova, and Giuseppe Giannaccare. "Non-Arteritic Anterior Ischemic Optic Neurop-

athy in an Otherwise Healthy Young Adult Patient Treated with Liraglutide and Semaglutide for Weight Loss: A Cautionary Tale." *International Medical Case Reports Journal* 18 (2025): 991–95.

38. American Diabetes Association Professional Practice Committee. "12. Retinopathy, Neuropathy, and Foot Care: Standards of Care in Diabetes—2025." *Diabetes Care* 48, suppl. 1 (2025): S252–65.

39. Akil, Handan, Jamie Burgess, Sarah Nevitt, Simon P. Harding, Uazman Alam, and Philip Burgess. "Early Worsening of Retinopathy in Type 1 and Type 2 Diabetes After Rapid Improvement in Glycemic Control: A Systematic Review." *Diabetes Therapy* 13, no. 1 (2022): 1–23.

40. Wang, Feiyu, Yinjun Mao, Hang Wang, Yiwei Liu, and Pinfang Huang. "Semaglutide and Diabetic Retinopathy Risk in Patients with Type 2 Diabetes Mellitus: A Meta-Analysis of Randomized Controlled Trials." *Clinical Drug Investigation* 42, no. 1 (2022): 17–28.

41. Heymsfield, Steven B., David S. Ludwig, Julia M. W. Wong et al. "Are Methods of Estimating Fat-Free Mass Loss with Energy-Restricted Diets Accurate?" *European Journal of Clinical Nutrition* 77, no. 5 (2023): 525–31.

42. Karakasis, Paschalis, Dimitrios Patoulias, Nikolaos Fragakis, and Christos, S. Mantzoros. "Effect of Glucagon-Like Peptide-1 Receptor Agonists and Co-Agonists on Body Composition: Systematic Review and Network Meta-Analysis." *Metabolism* 164 (2025): 156113.

43. Hopkins, Mark, Catherine Gibbons, and John Blundell. "Fat-Free Mass and Resting Metabolic Rate Are Determinants of Energy Intake: Implications for a Theory of Appetite Control." *Philosophical Transactions of the Royal Society B: Biological Sciences* 378, no. 1885 (2023): 20220213.

44. Martins, Catia, Jessica Roekenes, Barbara A. Gower, and Gary R. Hunter. "Metabolic Adaptation Is Associated with Less Weight and Fat Mass Loss in Response to Low-Energy Diets." *Nutrition & Metabolism* 18 (2021): 60, https://www.ncbi.nlm.nih.gov/pmc/articles/PMC8196522/.

45. Nunes, Everson A., Lauren Colenso-Semple, Sean R. McKellar et al. "Systematic Review and Meta-Analysis of Protein Intake to Support Muscle Mass and Function in Healthy Adults." *Journal of Cachexia, Sarcopenia and Muscle* 13, no. 2 (2022): 795–810.

46. Hudson, Joshua L., Yu Wang, Robert E. Bergia III, and Wayne W. Campbell. "Protein Intake Greater than the RDA Differentially Influences Whole-Body Lean Mass Responses to Purposeful Catabolic and Anabolic Stressors: A Systematic Review and Meta-Analysis." *Advances in Nutrition* 11, no. 3 (2020): 548–58.

47. Yazdanpanah, Zeinab, Sara Beigrezaei, Sahar Mohseni-Takalloo et al. "Does Exercise Affect Bone Mineral Density and Content When Added to a Calorie-Restricted Diet? A Systematic Review and Meta-Analysis of Controlled Clinical Trials." *Osteoporosis International* 33, no. 2 (2022): 339–54.

48. Joshi, Girish P., Teresa LaMasters, and Tammy L. Kindel. "Preprocedure Care of Patients on Glucagon-Like Peptide-1 Receptor Agonists: A Multisociety Clinical Practice Guidance." *Anesthesiology* 141, no. 6 (2024): 1208–9.

49. Kindel, Tammy L., Andrew Y. Wang, Anupama Wadhwa et al. "Multisociety Clinical Practice Guidance for the Safe Use of Glucagon-Like Peptide-1 Receptor Agonists in the Perioperative Period." *Surgery for Obesity and Related Diseases* 20, no. 12 (2024): 1183–86.

50. Manoharan, Senthil V. R. R., and Rohit Madan. "GLP-1 Agonists Can Affect Mood: A Case of Worsened Depression on Ozempic (Semaglutide)." *Innovations in Clinical Neuroscience* 21, nos. 4–6 (2024): 25–26.

51. Wang, William, Nora D. Volkow, Nathan A. Berger, Pamela B. Davis, David C. Kaelber, and Rong Xu. "Association of Semaglutide with Risk of Suicidal Ideation in a Real-World Cohort." *Nature Medicine* 30, no. 1 (2024): 168–76.

52. Di Stefano, Ramona, Lorenzo V. Rindi, Valentina Baldini et al. "Glucagon-Like Peptide-1 Receptor Agonists, Dual GIP/GLP-1 Receptor Agonist Tirzepatide and Suicidal Ideation and Behavior: A Systematic Review of Clinical Studies and Pharmacovigilance Reports." *Diabetes and Metabolic Syndrome* 19, no. 4 (2025): 103238. doi:10.1016/j.dsx.2025.103238.

53. Arillotta, Davide, Giuseppe Floresta, Amira Guirguis et al. "GLP-1 Receptor Agonists and Related Mental Health Issues: Insights from a Range of Social Media Platforms Using a Mixed-Methods Approach." *Brain Sciences* 13, no. 11 (2023): 1503.

54. Haggerty, Treah, Patricia Dekeseredy, Joanna Bailey, Abigail Cowher, Adam Baus, and Laura Davisson. "Navigating Coverage:

A Qualitative Study Exploring the Perceived Impact of an Insurance Company Policy to Discontinue Coverage of Antiobesity Medication." *Obesity Pillars* 11 (2024): 100120, https://www.ncbi.nlm.nih.gov/pmc/articles/PMC11332068/.

55. Waldrop, Stephanie W., Veronica R. Johnson, and Fatima Cody Stanford. "Inequalities in the Provision of GLP-1 Receptor Agonists for the Treatment of Obesity." *Nature Medicine* 30, no. 1 (2024): 22–25.

56. Butuca, Anca, Carmen Maximiliana Dobrea, Anca Maria Arseniu et al. "An Assessment of Semaglutide Safety Based on Real World Data: From Popularity to Spontaneous Reporting in EudraVigilance Database." *Biomedicines* 12, no. 5 (2024): 1124, https://www.ncbi.nlm.nih.gov/pmc/articles/PMC11117978/.

57. Berg, Sara, Hannah Stickle, Suzanne J. Rose, and Eric C. Nemec. "Discontinuing Glucagon-Like Peptide-1 Receptor Agonists and Body Habitus: A Systematic Review and Meta-Analysis." *Obesity Reviews* 26, no. 8 (2025): e13929.

58. Denny, Olivia, Jeffrey Baron, and Nicole P. Albanese. "Navigating Glucagon-Like Peptide Receptor Agonist Reinitiation amid Access Barriers: An Adverse Drug Event Case Report." *Journal of Pharmacy Practice* 37, no. 6 (2024): 1410–13.

59. Gleason, Patrick P., Benjamin Y. Urick, Landon Z. Marshall, Nicholas Friedlander, Yang Qiu, and R. Scott Leslie. "Real-World Persistence and Adherence to Glucagon-Like Peptide-1 Receptor Agonists Among Obese Commercially Insured Adults Without Diabetes." *Journal of Managed Care & Specialty Pharmacy* 30, no. 8 (2024): 860–67.

60. Kim, Ju Young. "Optimal Diet Strategies for Weight Loss and Weight Loss Maintenance." *Journal of Obesity & Metabolic Syndrome* 30, no. 1 (2021): 20–31, https://www.ncbi.nlm.nih.gov/pmc/articles/PMC8017325/.

61. Nreu, Besmir, Ilaria Dicembrini, Federico Tinti, Edoardo Mannucci, and Matteo Monami. "Pancreatitis and Pancreatic Cancer in Patients with Type 2 Diabetes Treated with Glucagon-Like Peptide-1 Receptor Agonists: An Updated Meta-Analysis of Randomized Controlled Trials." *Minerva Endocrinology* 48, no. 2 (2023): 206–13.

62. Kapoor, Ishani, Swara M. Sarvepalli, David D'Alessio, Dilraj S. Grewal, and Majda Hadziahmetovic. "GLP-1 Receptor Agonists

and Diabetic Retinopathy: A Meta-Analysis of Randomized Clinical Trials." *Survey of Ophthalmology* 68, no. 6 (2023): 1071–83.

63. Look, Michelle, Julia P. Dunn, Robert F. Kushner et al. "Body Composition Changes During Weight Reduction with Tirzepatide in the SURMOUNT-1 Study of Adults with Obesity or Overweight." *Diabetes, Obesity and Metabolism* 27, no. 5 (2025): 2720–29.

Chapter 3: The Origin Story of Akker

1. Cavaillon, Jean-Marc, and Sandra Legout. "Centenary of the Death of Élie Metchnikoff: A Visionary and an Outstanding Team Leader." *Microbes and Infection* 18, no. 10 (2016): 577–94.

2. Underhill, David M., Siamon Gordon, Beat A. Imhof, Gabriel Núñez, and Philippe Bousso. "Élie Metchnikoff (1845–1916): Celebrating 100 Years of Cellular Immunology and Beyond." *Nature Reviews Immunology* 16, no. 10 (2016): 651–56.

3. Kaufmann, Stefan H. E. "Immunology's Foundation: The 100-Year Anniversary of the Nobel Prize to Paul Ehrlich and Élie Metchnikoff." *Nature Immunology* 9, no. 7 (2008): 705–12.

4. Calvanese, Chiara Maria, Francesco Villani, Danilo Ercolini, and Francesca De Filippis. "Postbiotics Versus Probiotics: Possible New Allies for Human Health." *Food Research International* 217 (2025): 116869.

5. Merkouris, Ermis, Theodora Mavroudi, Daniil Miliotas et al. "Probiotics' Effects in the Treatment of Anxiety and Depression: A Comprehensive Review of 2014–2023 Clinical Trials." *Microorganisms* 12, no. 2 (2024): 411.

6. Aalipanah, Erfaneh, Moein Askarpour, Mohammad Hadi Eskandari et al. "Comparing the Effects of Yogurt Containing *Akkermansia muciniphila* Postbiotic with Yogurt Containing *Lactobacillus rhamnosus* Postbiotic on Body Composition, Biochemical Indices, Appetite, and Depression Scores in Overweight or Obese Adults: A Randomized, Double-Blind, Controlled Clinical Trial." *Clinical Nutrition ESPEN* 68 (2025): 438–46.

7. Yang, Xinyu, Xiaoye Cheng, Yiting Tang et al. "The Role of Type 1 Interferons in Coagulation Induced by Gram-Negative Bacteria." *Blood* 135, no. 14 (2020): 1087–100.

8. Bindels, Laure B., Nathalie M. Delzenne, Patrice D. Cani, and Jens Walter. "Towards a More Comprehensive Concept for Prebi-

otics." *Nature Reviews Gastroenterology & Hepatology* 12, no. 5 (2015): 303–10.

9. Nazarinejad, Zahra, Roghayeh Molani-Gol, Leila Roozbeh Nasiraie, and Vahideh Ebrahimzadeh-Attari. "Postbiotics as a Novel Intervention for Obesity Management and Improving Metabolic Parameters: A Systematic Review and Meta-Analysis of Animal Studies." *Journal of Translational Medicine* 23, no. 1 (2025): 913.

10. Lloyd-Price, Jason, Cesar Arze, Ashwin N. Ananthakrishnan et al. "Multi-Omics of the Gut Microbial Ecosystem in Inflammatory Bowel Diseases." *Nature* 569, no. 7758 (2019): 655–62.

11. Ioannou, Athanasia, Maryse D. Berkhout, Sharon Y. Geerlings, and Clara Belzer. "*Akkermansia muciniphila*: Biology, Microbial Ecology, Host Interactions and Therapeutic Potential." *Nature Reviews: Microbiology* 23, no. 3 (2025): 162–77.

12. De Vos, Willem M. "Microbe Profile: *Akkermansia muciniphila*: A Conserved Intestinal Symbiont That Acts as the Gatekeeper of Our Mucosa." *Microbiology* 163, no. 5 (2017): 646–48.

13. De Vos, Willem M., Herbert Tilg, Matthias Van Hul, and Patrice D. Cani. "Gut Microbiome and Health: Mechanistic Insights." *Gut* 71, no. 5 (2022): 1020–32.

14. Tidjani Alou, Maryam, Sabrina Naud, Saber Khelaifia, Marion Bonnet, Jean-Christophe Lagier, and Didier Raoult. "State of the Art in the Culture of the Human Microbiota: New Interests and Strategies." *Clinical Microbiology Reviews* 34, no. 1 (2020): e00129-19.

15. Barlow, Jacob T., Gabriela Leite, Anna E. Romano et al. "Quantitative Sequencing Clarifies the Role of Disruptor Taxa, Oral Microbiota, and Strict Anaerobes in the Human Small-Intestine Microbiome." *Microbiome* 9, no. 1 (2021): 214.

16. Konjar, Špela, Miha Pavšič, and Marc Veldhoen. "Regulation of Oxygen Homeostasis at the Intestinal Epithelial Barrier Site." *International Journal of Molecular Sciences* 22, no. 17 (2021): 9170.

17. Wang, Rui, Guoming Zhang, Xiaoya Wang, Zefeng Xing, Zhen Li, and Lixiang Li. "Effect of Bacillus Coagulans BC99 Supplementation on Body Weight and Gut Microbiota in Overweight and Obese Individual: A Randomized, Double-Blind, Placebo-Controlled Study." *Frontiers in Nutrition* 12 (2025), https://www.frontiersin.org/journals/nutrition/articles/10.3389/fnut.2025.1542145/full.

18. Gasaly, Naschla, Marcela A. Hermoso, and Martín Gotteland. "Butyrate and the Fine-Tuning of Colonic Homeostasis: Implication for Inflammatory Bowel Diseases." *International Journal of Molecular Sciences* 22, no. 6 (2021): 3061.

19. Gasaly, Naschla, Paul de Vos, and Marcela A. Hermoso. "Impact of Bacterial Metabolites on Gut Barrier Function and Host Immunity: A Focus on Bacterial Metabolism and Its Relevance for Intestinal Inflammation." *Frontiers in Immunology* 12 (2021): 658354.

20. Zhang, Zhan, Xinyue Wu, Shuyuan Cao et al. "Caffeic Acid Ameliorates Colitis in Association with Increased *Akkermansia* Population in the Gut Microbiota of Mice." *Oncotarget* 7, no. 22 (2016): 31790–99.

21. Davey, Lauren E., Per N. Malkus, Max Villa et al. "A Genetic System for *Akkermansia muciniphila* Reveals a Role for Mucin Foraging in Gut Colonization and Host Sterol Biosynthesis Gene Expression." *Nature Microbiology* 8, no. 8 (2023): 1450–67.

22. Paone, Paola, and Patrice D. Cani. "Mucus Barrier, Mucins and Gut Microbiota: The Expected Slimy Partners?" *Gut* 69, no. 12 (2020): 2232–43.

23. Belzer, Clara, Loo Wee Chia, Steven Aalvink et al. "Microbial Metabolic Networks at the Mucus Layer Lead to Diet-Independent Butyrate and Vitamin B12 Production by Intestinal Symbionts." *mBio* 8, no. 5 (2017): e00770-17.

24. Fernandes Rodrigues, Vanessa, Jefferson Elias-Oliveira, Ítalo Sousa Pereira et al. "*Akkermansia muciniphila* and Gut Immune System: A Good Friendship That Attenuates Inflammatory Bowel Disease, Obesity, and Diabetes." *Frontiers in Immunology* 13 (2022): 934695.

25. Karcher, Nicolai, Eleonora Nigro, Michal Punčochář et al. "Genomic Diversity and Ecology of Human-Associated *Akkermansia* Species in the Gut Microbiome Revealed by Extensive Metagenomic Assembly." *Genome Biology* 22, no. 1 (2021): 209.

26. Hansson, Gunnar C. "Role of Mucus Layers in Gut Infection and Inflammation." *Current Opinion in Microbiology* 15, no. 1 (2012): 57–62.

27. Everard, Amandine, Clara Belzer, Lucie Geurts et al. "Cross-Talk Between *Akkermansia muciniphila* and Intestinal

Epithelium Controls Diet-Induced Obesity." *Proceedings of the National Academy of Sciences of the United States of America* 110, no. 22 (2013): 9066–71.

28. Otani, Tetsuhisa, and Mikio Furuse. "Tight Junction Structure and Function Revisited." *Trends in Cell Biology* 30, no. 10 (2020): 805–17.

29. Ashrafian, Fatemeh, Ava Behrouzi, Arefeh Shahriary et al. "Comparative Study of Effect of *Akkermansia muciniphila* and Its Extracellular Vesicles on Toll-Like Receptors and Tight Junction." *Gastroenterology and Hepatology from Bed to Bench* 12, no. 2 (2019): 163–68.

30. Gao, Fangfang, Canyu Cheng, Runwei Li, Zongcun Chen, Ke Tang, and Guankui Du. "The Role of *Akkermansia muciniphila* in Maintaining Health: A Bibliometric Study." *Frontiers in Medicine* (2025), https://www.frontiersin.org/journals/medicine/articles/10.3389/fmed.2025.1484656/full.

31. Wang, Junchao, Wenjuan Xu, Rongjuan Wang, Rongrong Cheng, Zhengquan Tangac, and Min Zhang. "The Outer Membrane Protein Amuc_1100 of *Akkermansia muciniphila* Promotes Intestinal 5-HT Biosynthesis and Extracellular Availability Through TLR2 Signalling." *Food & Function* 12, no. 8 (2021): 3597–610.

32. Maślak, Ewelina, Wojciech Kupczyk, Viorica Railean, Paweł Pomastowski, Marek Jackowski, and Bogusław Buszewski. "Viability Study of Clinical Bacterial Strains by Capillary Electrophoresis and Flow Cytometry Approaches." *Electrophoresis* 43, no. 20 (2022): 2005–13.

33. Dao, Maria Carlota, Amandine Everard, Judith Aron-Wisnewsky et al. "*Akkermansia muciniphila* and Improved Metabolic Health During a Dietary Intervention in Obesity: Relationship with Gut Microbiome Richness and Ecology." *Gut* 65, no. 3 (2016): 426–36.

34. Cani, Patrice D., Clara Depommier, Muriel Derrien, Amandine Everard, and Willem M. de Vos. "*Akkermansia muciniphila*: Paradigm for Next-Generation Beneficial Microorganisms." *Nature Reviews Gastroenterology & Hepatology* 19, no. 10 (2022): 625–37.

35. Bosello, Ottavio, and Maria Pia Donataccio. "Obesity Paradox." *Eating and Weight Disorders* 18, no. 4 (2013): 447–48.

36. Depommier, Clara, Amandine Everard, Céline Druart et al. "Supplementation with *Akkermansia muciniphila* in Overweight

and Obese Human Volunteers: A Proof-of-Concept Exploratory Study." *Nature Medicine* 25, no. 7 (2019): 1096–103.

37. Ioannou, Athanasia, Maryse D. Berkhout, Sharon Y. Geerlings, and Clara Belzer. "*Akkermansia muciniphila*: Biology, Microbial Ecology, Host Interactions and Therapeutic Potential." *Nature Reviews Microbiology* 23, no. 3 (2025): 162–77.

38. Vallianou, Natalia, Gerasimos Socrates Christodoulatos, Irene Karampela et al. "Understanding the Role of the Gut Microbiome and Microbial Metabolites in Non-Alcoholic Fatty Liver Disease: Current Evidence and Perspectives." *Biomolecules* 12, no. 1 (2021): 56.

39. Rodríguez-Daza, María Carolina, and Willem M. de Vos. "Polyphenols as Drivers of a Homeostatic Gut Microecology and Immuno-Metabolic Traits of *Akkermansia muciniphila*: From Mouse to Man." *International Journal of Molecular Sciences* 24, no. 1 (2022): 45.

40. Giongo, Adriana, Kelsey A. Gano, David B. Crabb et al. "Toward Defining the Autoimmune Microbiome for Type 1 Diabetes." *ISME Journal* 5, no. 1 (2011): 82–91.

41. Xu, Yu, Ning Wang, Hor-Yue Tan, Sha Li, Cheng Zhang, and Yibin Feng. "Function of *Akkermansia muciniphila* in Obesity: Interactions with Lipid Metabolism, Immune Response and Gut Systems." *Frontiers in Microbiology* 11 (2020): 219.

42. Zhou, Qi, Yanfeng Zhang, Xiaoxia Wang et al. "Gut Bacteria *Akkermansia* Is Associated with Reduced Risk of Obesity: Evidence from the American Gut Project." *Nutrition & Metabolism* 17 (2020): 90.

43. Matson, Vyara, Jessica Fessler, Riyue Bao et al. "The Commensal Microbiome Is Associated with Anti-PD-1 Efficacy in Metastatic Melanoma Patients." *Science* 359, no. 6371 (2018): 104–8.

44. Huang, Zhiqiang, Kun Liu, Wenwen Ma, Dezhi Li, Tianlu Mo, and Qing Liu. "The Gut Microbiome in Human Health and Disease—Where Are We and Where Are We Going? A Bibliometric Analysis." *Frontiers in Microbiology* 13 (2022): 1018594.

45. Salminen, Seppo, Maria Carmen Collado, Akihito Endo et al. "The International Scientific Association of Probiotics and Prebiotics (ISAPP) Consensus Statement on the Definition and Scope of Postbiotics." *Nature Reviews Gastroenterology & Hepatology* 18, no. 9 (2021): 649–67.

46. Ropot, Anastasiia V., Andrei M. Karamzin, and Oleg V. Sergeyev. "Cultivation of the Next-Generation Probiotic *Akkermansia muciniphila*, Methods of Its Safe Delivery to the Intestine, and Factors Contributing to Its Growth In Vivo." *Current Microbiology* 77, no. 8 (2020): 1363–72.

47. Qu, Linkai, Jiaxuan He, Ting Xu et al. "Therapeutic Effects of Pasteurized *Akkermansia muciniphila* on Metabolic and Behavioral Dysregulation in a Zebrafish Model of Type 2 Diabetes Mellitus Comorbid with Depression." *Journal of Functional Foods* 129 (2025): 106848.

48. Barbosa, Joana Cristina, Diana Almeida, Daniela Machado et al. "Spray-Drying Encapsulation of the Live Biotherapeutic Candidate *Akkermansia muciniphila* DSM 22959 to Survive Aerobic Storage." *Pharmaceuticals (Basel)* 15, no. 5 (2022): 628.

49. Li, Zhitao, Guoao Hu, Li Zhu et al. "Study of Growth, Metabolism, and Morphology of *Akkermansia muciniphila* with an In Vitro Advanced Bionic Intestinal Reactor." *BMC Microbiology* 21, no. 1 (2021): 61.

50. Bae, Munhyung, Chelsi D. Cassilly, Xiaoxi Liu et al. "*Akkermansia muciniphila* Phospholipid Induces Homeostatic Immune Responses." *Nature* 608, no. 7921 (2022): 168–73.

51. Özkul, Ceren, Meltem Yalınay, and Tarkan Karakan. "Islamic Fasting Leads to an Increased Abundance of *Akkermansia muciniphila* and *Bacteroides fragilis* Group: A Preliminary Study on Intermittent Fasting." *Turkish Journal of Gastroenterology* 30, no. 12 (2019): 1030–35.

52. Rudrapal, Mithun, Shubham J. Khairnar, Johra Khan et al. "Dietary Polyphenols and Their Role in Oxidative Stress-Induced Human Diseases: Insights into Protective Effects, Antioxidant Potentials and Mechanism(s) of Action." *Frontiers in Pharmacology* 13 (2022): 806470.

53. Roopchand, Diana E., Rachel N. Carmody, Peter Kuhn et al. "Dietary Polyphenols Promote Growth of the Gut Bacterium *Akkermansia muciniphila* and Attenuate High-Fat Diet-Induced Metabolic Syndrome." *Diabetes* 64, no. 8 (2015): 2847–58.

54. Haak, Bastiaan W., Eric R. Littmann, Jean-Luc Chaubard et al. "Impact of Gut Colonization with Butyrate-Producing Microbiota on Respiratory Viral Infection Following Allo-HCT." *Blood* 131, no. 26 (2018): 2978–86.

55. Ganesh, Bhanu Priya, Robert Klopfleisch, Gunnar Loh, and Michael Blaut. "Commensal *Akkermansia muciniphila* Exacerbates Gut Inflammation in *Salmonella Typhimurium*-Infected Gnotobiotic Mice." *PLoS One* 8, no. 9 (2013): e74963.

56. Wang, Fei, Kuntai Cai, Qiuxiang Xiao, Lihua He, Lu Xie, and Zhiping Liu. "*Akkermansia muciniphila* Administration Exacerbated the Development of Colitis-Associated Colorectal Cancer in Mice." *Journal of Cancer* 13, no. 1 (2022): 124–33.

57. Noori, Pegah, Fattah Sotoodehnejadnematalahi, Pooneh Rahimi, and Seyed Davar Siadat. "*Akkermansia muciniphila* and Its Extracellular Vesicles Affect Endocannabinoid System in In Vitro Model." *Digestion* 106, no. 4 (2025): 338–48.

58. Ghaderi, Farinaz, Fattah Sotoodehnejadnematalahi, Zahra Hajebrahimi, Abolfazl Fateh, and Seyed Davar Siadat. "Effects of Active, Inactive, and Derivatives of *Akkermansia muciniphila* on the Expression of the Endocannabinoid System and PPARs Genes." *Scientific Reports* 12, no. 1 (2022): 10031.

59. Yaghoubfar, Rezvan, Ava Behrouzi, Fatemeh Ashrafian et al. "Modulation of Serotonin Signaling/Metabolism by *Akkermansia muciniphila* and Its Extracellular Vesicles Through the Gut-Brain Axis in Mice." *Scientific Reports* 10, no. 1 (2020): 22119.

Chapter 4: Colonocytes, Gut Gems, and Your Gut Barrier

1. Nazarinejad, Zahra, Roghayeh Molani-Gol, Leila Roozbeh Nasiraie, and Vahideh Ebrahimzadeh-Attari. "Postbiotics as a Novel Intervention for Obesity Management and Improving Metabolic Parameters: A Systematic Review and Meta-Analysis of Animal Studies." *Journal of Translational Medicine* 23, no. 1 (2025): 913.

2. Gasaly, Naschla, Marcela A. Hermoso, and Martín Gotteland. "Butyrate and the Fine-Tuning of Colonic Homeostasis: Implication for Inflammatory Bowel Diseases." *International Journal of Molecular Sciences* 22, no. 6 (2021): 3061.

3. Salvi, Pooja, S., and Robert A. Cowles. "Butyrate and the Intestinal Epithelium: Modulation of Proliferation and Inflammation in Homeostasis and Disease." *Cells* 10, no. 7 (2021): 1775.

4. Li, Zhitao, Guoao Hu, Li Zhu et al. "Study of Growth, Metabolism, and Morphology of *Akkermansia muciniphila* with an In Vitro Advanced Bionic Intestinal Reactor." *BMC Microbiology* 21, no. 1 (2021): 61.

5. Liu, Pinyi, Yanbing Wang, Ge Yang et al. "The Role of Short-Chain Fatty Acids in Intestinal Barrier Function, Inflammation, Oxidative Stress, and Colonic Carcinogenesis." *Pharmacological Research* 165 (2021): 105420.

6. Hodgkinson, Kendra, Faiha El Abbar, Peter Dobranowski et al. "Butyrate's Role in Human Health and the Current Progress Towards Its Clinical Application to Treat Gastrointestinal Disease." Clinical Nutrition 42, no. 2 (2023): 61–75.

7. Recharla, Neeraja, Ramasatyaveni Geesala, and Xuan-Zheng Shi. "Gut Microbial Metabolite Butyrate and Its Therapeutic Role in Inflammatory Bowel Disease: A Literature Review." *Nutrients* 15, no. 10 (2023): 2275.

8. Savage, Hannah P., Derek J. Bays, Connor R. Tiffany et al. "Epithelial Hypoxia Maintains Colonization Resistance Against *Candida albicans*." *Cell Host and Microbe* 32, no. 7 (2024): 1103–13.

9. Fagundes, Raphael R., Saskia C. Belt, Barbara M. Bakker et al. "Beyond Butyrate: Microbial Fiber Metabolism Supporting Colonic Epithelial Homeostasis." *Trends in Microbiology* 32, no. 2 (2024): 178–89.

10. Calvanese, Chiara Maria, Francesco Villani, Danilo Ercolini, and Francesca De Filippis. "Postbiotics Versus Probiotics: Possible New Allies for Human Health." *Food Research International* 217 (2025): 116869.

11. Bayer Christiansen, Charlotte, Maria Buur Nordskov Gabe, Berit Svendsen, Lars Ove Dragsted, Mette Marie Rosenkilde, and Jens Juul Holst. "The Impact of Short-Chain Fatty Acids on GLP-1 and PYY Secretion from the Isolated Perfused Rat Colon." *American Journal of Physiology: Gastrointestinal and Liver Physiology* 315, no. 1 (2018): G53–65.

12. Mann, Elizabeth R., Ying Ka Lam, and Holm H. Uhlig. "Short-Chain Fatty Acids: Linking Diet, the Microbiome and Immunity." *Nature Reviews: Immunology* 24, no. 8 (2024): 577–95.

13. Ojo, Omorogieva, Qian-Qian Feng, Osarhumwese Osaretin Ojo, and Xiao-Hua Wang. "The Role of Dietary Fibre in Modulating Gut Microbiota Dysbiosis in Patients with Type 2 Diabetes: A Systematic Review and Meta-Analysis of Randomised Controlled Trials." *Nutrients* 12, no. 11 (2020): 3239.

14. Luis, Ana S., and Gunnar C. Hansson. "Intestinal Mucus and Their Glycans: A Habitat for Thriving Microbiota." *Cell Host and Microbe* 31, no. 7 (2023): 1087–100.

15. Pietrzak, Bernadeta, Katarzyna Tomela, Agnieszka Olejnik-Schmidt, Andrzej Mackiewicz, and Marcin Schmidt. "Secretory IgA in Intestinal Mucosal Secretions as an Adaptive Barrier against Microbial Cells." *International Journal of Molecular Sciences* 21, no. 23 (2020): 9254.

16. Pral, Laís P., José L. Fachi, Renan O. Corrêa, Marco Colonna, and Marco A. R. Vinolo. "Hypoxia and HIF-1 as Key Regulators of Gut Microbiota and Host Interactions." *Trends in Immunology* 42, no. 7 (2021): 604–21.

17. Zheng, Leon, Caleb J. Kelly, and Sean P. Colgan. "Physiologic Hypoxia and Oxygen Homeostasis in the Healthy Intestine. A Review in the Theme: Cellular Responses to Hypoxia." *American Journal of Physiology: Cell Physiology* 309, no. 6 (2015): C350–360.

18. Konjar Š, Pavšič M, Veldhoen M. Regulation of Oxygen Homeostasis at the Intestinal Epithelial Barrier Site. Int J Mol Sci. 2021 Aug 25; 22(17): 9170.

19. Byndloss, Mariana X., Erin E. Olsan, Fabian Rivera-Chávez et al. "Microbiota-Activated PPAR-γ Signaling Inhibits Dysbiotic Enterobacteriaceae Expansion." *Science* 357, no. 6351 (2017): 570–75.

20. Gao, Fangfang, Canyu Cheng, Runwei Li, Zongcun Chen, Ke Tang, and Guankui Du. "The Role of *Akkermansia muciniphila* in Maintaining Health: A Bibliometric Study." *Frontiers in Medicine*, vol. 12, February 3, 2025, https://www.frontiersin.org/journals/medicine/articles/10.3389/fmed.2025.1484656/full

21. Mohammad, Shireen, and Christoph Thiemermann. "Role of Metabolic Endotoxemia in Systemic Inflammation and Potential Interventions." *Frontiers in Immunology* 11, (2020): 594150.

22. Khoshbin, Katayoun, and Michael Camilleri. "Effects of Dietary Components on Intestinal Permeability in Health and Disease." *American Journal of Physiology: Gastrointestinal and Liver Physiology* 319, no. 5 (2020): G589–608.

23. Liu, Huixia, Chun Zhang, and Jing Xiong. "Pathological Connections Between Nonalcoholic Fatty Liver Disease and Chronic Kidney Disease." *Kidney Diseases* 8, no. 6 (2022): 458–65.

Chapter 5: The Seed-Oil Catastrophe: How Seed Oils Changed Your Gut's Ecosystem

1. Blasbalg, Tanya L., Joseph R. Hibbeln, Christopher E. Ramsden, Sharon F. Majchrzak, and Robert R. Rawlings. "Changes in Consumption of Omega-3 and Omega-6 Fatty Acids in the United States during the 20th Century." American Journal Clinical Nutrition 93, no. 5 (2011): 950–62.

2. Mousavi, Seyed Mohammad, Yahya Jalilpiran, Elmira Karimi et al. "Dietary Intake of Linoleic Acid, Its Concentrations, and the Risk of Type 2 Diabetes: A Systematic Review and Dose-Response Meta-Analysis of Prospective Cohort Studies." *Diabetes Care* 44, no. 9 (2021): 2173–81.

3. Yang, Li, Li-Mian Cao, Xiao-Ju Zhang, and Bo Chu. "Targeting Ferroptosis as a Vulnerability in Pulmonary Diseases." *Cell Death and Disease* 13, no. 7 (2022): 649.

4. Schulze, Matthias B. "Dietary Linoleic Acid: Will Modifying Dietary Fat Quality Reduce the Risk of Type 2 Diabetes?" *Diabetes Care* 44, no. 9 (2021): 1913–5.

5. Zhang, Yifei, Ruixin Liu, Yufei Chen et al. "*Akkermansia muciniphila* Supplementation in Patients with Overweight/Obese Type 2 Diabetes: Efficacy Depends On Its Baseline Levels in the Gut." *Cell Metabolism* 37, no. 3 (2025): 592–605.

6. Shrestha, Nirajan, Simone L. Sleep, James S. M. Cuffe et al. "Role of Omega-6 and Omega-3 Fatty Acids in Fetal Programming." Clinical and Experimental Pharmacology and Physiology 47, no. 5 (2020): 907–15.

7. You, Jie, Wu Liu, Yuxiong Huange et al. "*Akkermansia muciniphila* PROBIO Ameliorates Overweight Via Gut Microbiota Modulation: A Randomized Controlled Trial." *Food Science and Human Wellness*, June 12, 2025, https://www.sciopen.com/article/10.26599/FSHW.2025.9250659.

8. Ganguly, Archan, Xuemei Han, Utpal Das et al. "Hsc70 Chaperone Activity Is Required for the Cytosolic Slow Axonal Transport of Synapsin." *Journal of Cell Biology* 216, no. 7 (2017): 2059–74.

9. Rohrhofer, Johanna, Benjamin Zwirzitz, Evelyne Selberherr, and Eva Untersmayr. "The Impact of Dietary Sphingolipids on Intestinal Microbiota and Gastrointestinal Immune Homeostasis." *Frontiers in Immunology* 12 (2021): 635704.

10. Chen, Yuwei, Yongbo She, Ruisan Zhang, Jieying Wang, Xiaohua Zhang, and Xingchun Gou. "Use of Starch-Based Fat Replacers in Foods as a Strategy to Reduce Dietary Intake of Fat and Risk of Metabolic Diseases." *Food Science and Nutrition* 8, no. 1 (2020): 16–22.

11. Wang, Rui, Guoming Zhang, Xiaoya Wang, Zefeng Xing, Zhen Li, and Lixiang Li. "Effect of Bacillus Coagulans BC99 Supplementation on Body Weight and Gut Microbiota in Overweight and Obese Individual: A Randomized, Double-Blind, Placebo-Controlled Study." *Frontiers in Nutrition* 12 (2025), https://www.frontiersin.org/journals/nutrition/articles/10.3389/fnut.2025.1542145/full.

12. Haddad, Yara K., Iju Shakya, Briana L. Moreland, Ramakrishna Kakara, and Gwen Bergen. "Injury Diagnosis and Affected Body Part for Nonfatal Fall-Related Injuries in Community-Dwelling Older Adults Treated in Emergency Departments." *Journal of Aging and Health* 32, no. 10 (2020): 1433–42.

13. Rhoads, Megan K., Slavina B. Goleva, William H. Beierwaltes, and Jeffrey L. Osborn. "Renal Vascular and Glomerular Pathologies Associated with Spontaneous Hypertension in the Nonhuman Primate *Chlorocebus aethiops sabaeus*." *American Journal of Physiology: Regulatory, Integrative, and Comparative Physiology* 313, no. 3 (2017): R211–8.

14. Kabagambe, Sandra, Benjamin Keller, James Becker et al. "Placental Mesenchymal Stromal Cells Seeded on Clinical Grade Extracellular Matrix Improve Ambulation in Ovine Myelomeningocele." *Journal of Pediatric Surgery* S0022-3468, no. 17 (2017): 30654–1.

15. Mericliler, Meric, Vera Kazakova, Diala Nicolas, Utkarsh H. Acharya, and Bertrand L. Jaber. "Improving Compliance with Appropriateness of Testing for Heparin-Induced Thrombocytopaenia: A Quality Improvement Report." *BMJ Open Quality* 11, no. 3 (2022): e001746.

16. Hall, Kevin D., Alexis Ayuketah, Robert Brychta et al. "Ultra-Processed Diets Cause Excess Calorie Intake and Weight Gain: An Inpatient Randomized Controlled Trial of Ad Libitum Food Intake." *Cell Metabolism* 30, no. 1 (2019): 67–77.

17. Ruiz de Alegría Puig, C., M. Macho Díaz, J. Agüero Balbín, and J. Calvo Montes. "First Case of *Arcobacter cryaerophilus* in Paediatric Age in Spain." *Revista Española de Quimioterapia: Publi-

cación Oficial de la Sociedad Española de Quimioterapia 34, no. 3 (2021): 259–60.

18. Emami, E. "COVID-19: Perspective of a Dean of Dentistry." *JDR Clinical and Translational Research* 5, no. 3 (2020): 211–3.

19. García-González, Aída, Joaquín Velasco, Leonardo Velasco, and M. Victoria Ruiz-Méndez. "Attempts of Physical Refining of Sterol-Rich Sunflower Press Oil to Obtain Minimally Processed Edible Oil." *Foods* 10, no. 8 (2021): 1901.

20. Lei, Lei, Jianan Zhang, Eric A. Decker, and Guodong Zhang. "Roles of Lipid Peroxidation-Derived Electrophiles in Pathogenesis of Colonic Inflammation and Colon Cancer." *Frontiers in Cell and Developmental Biology* 9 (2021): 665591.

21. Milkovic, Lidija, Neven Zarkovic, Zlatko Marusic, Kamelija Zarkovic, and Morana Jaganjac. "The 4-Hydroxynonenal-Protein Adducts and Their Biological Relevance: Are Some Proteins Preferred Targets?" *Antioxidants* 12, no. 4 (2023): 856.

22. Pral, Laís P., José L. Fachi, Renan O. Corrêa, Marco Colonna, and Marco A. R. Vinolo. "Hypoxia and HIF-1 as Key Regulators of Gut Microbiota and Host Interactions." *Trends in Immunology* 42, no. 7 (2021): 604–21.

23. Zhang, Jianan, Xijing Chen, Ran Yang et al. "Thermally Processed Oil Exaggerates Colonic Inflammation and Colitis-Associated Colon Tumorigenesis in Mice." *Cancer Prevention Research* 12, no. 11 (2019): 741–50.

24. Wang, Yuxin, Weicang Wang, Haixia Yang, Derek Shao, Xinfeng Zhao, and Guodong Zhang. "Intraperitoneal Injection of 4-Hydroxynonenal (4-HNE), a Lipid Peroxidation Product, Exacerbates Colonic Inflammation Through Activation of Toll-Like Receptor 4 Signaling." *Free Radical Biology and Medicine* 131 (2019): 237–42.

25. Yoo, Woongjae, Jacob K. Zieba, Nora J. Foegeding et al. "High-Fat Diet-Induced Colonocyte Dysfunction Escalates Microbiota-Derived Trimethylamine N-Oxide." *Science* 373, no. 6556 (2021): 813–18.

26. Gonçalves, Pedro, Inês Gregório, Telmo A. Catarino, and Fátima Martel. "The Effect of Oxidative Stress Upon the Intestinal Epithelial Uptake of Butyrate." *European Journal of Pharmacology* 699, nos. 1–3 (2013): 88–100.

27. Salvi, Pooja S., and Robert A. Cowles. "Butyrate and the Intestinal Epithelium: Modulation of Proliferation and Inflammation in Homeostasis and Disease." *Cells* 10, no. 7 (2021): 1775.

28. El-Sayed, Hemat S., Aalaa S. Saad, Wesam A. Tawfik et al. "The Role of Turmeric and Black Pepper Oil Nanoemulsion in Attenuating Cytokine Storm Triggered by Duck Hepatitis A Virus Type I (DHAV-I)-Induced Infection in Ducklings." *Poultry Science* 103, no. 3 (2024): 103404.

29. Byndloss, Mariana X., Erin E. Olsan, Fabian Rivera-Chávez et al. "Microbiota-Activated PPAR-Γ Signaling Inhibits Dysbiotic Enterobacteriaceae Expansion." *Science* 357, no. 6351 (2017): 570–75.

30. Sun Penghao, Mengli Wang, Yong-Xin Liu et al. "High-Fat Diet-Disturbed Gut Microbiota-Colonocyte Interactions Contribute to Dysregulating Peripheral Tryptophan-Kynurenine Metabolism." *Microbiome* 11, no. 1 (2023): 154.

31. Mishra, Animesh A., and Andrew Y. Koh. "Breathe and Bloom: Gut Hypoxia Limits *C. albicans* Growth." *Cell Host and Microbe* 32, no. 7 (2024): 1041–43.

32. Litvak, Yael, Mariana X. Byndloss, and Andreas J. Bäumler. "Colonocyte Metabolism Shapes the Gut Microbiota." *Science* 362, no. 6418 (2018): eaat9076.

33. Merra, Giuseppe, Annalisa Noce, Giulia Marrone et al. "Influence of Mediterranean Diet on Human Gut Microbiota." *Nutrients* 13, no. 1 (2020): 7.

34. McQuade, Jennifer L., Gabriel O. Ologun, Reetakshi Arora, and Jennifer A. Wargo. "Gut Microbiome Modulation Via Fecal Microbiota Transplant to Augment Immunotherapy in Patients with Melanoma or Other Cancers." *Current Oncology Reports* 22, no. 7 (2020): 74.

35. Liu, Pinyi, Yanbing Wang, Ge Yang et al. "The Role of Short-Chain Fatty Acids in Intestinal Barrier Function, Inflammation, Oxidative Stress, and Colonic Carcinogenesis." *Pharmacological Research* 165 (2021): 105420.

36. Hanning, Nikita, Adam L. Edwinson, Hannah Ceuleers et al. "Intestinal Barrier Dysfunction in Irritable Bowel Syndrome: A Systematic Review." *Therapeutic Advances in Gastroenterology* 14 (2021): 1756284821993586.

37. García-Montero, Cielo, Oscar Fraile-Martínez, Ana M. Gómez-Lahoz et al. "Nutritional Components in Western Diet Versus Mediterranean Diet at the Gut Microbiota-Immune System Interplay. Implications for Health and Disease." *Nutrients* 13, no. 2 (2021): 699.

38. Singh, Vineet, GyuDae Lee, HyunWoo Son et al. "Butyrate Producers, 'The Sentinel of Gut': Their Intestinal Significance with and Beyond Butyrate, and Prospective Use as Microbial Therapeutics." *Frontiers in Microbiology* 13 (2022): 1103836.

39. Hou, Huiqin, Danfeng Chen, Kexin Zhang et al. "Gut Microbiota-Derived Short-Chain Fatty Acids and Colorectal Cancer: Ready for Clinical Translation?" *Cancer Letters* 526 (2022): 225–35.

40. Qu, Linkai, Jiaxuan He, Ting Xu et al. "Therapeutic Effects Of Pasteurized *Akkermansia muciniphila* on Metabolic and Behavioral Dysregulation in a Zebrafish Model of Type 2 Diabetes Mellitus Comorbid with Depression." *Journal of Functional Foods* 129 (2025): 106848.

41. Hijová, Emília, Izabela Bertková, and Jana Štofilová. "Incorporating Postbiotics into Intervention for Managing Obesity." *International Journal of Molecular Sciences* 26, no. 11 (2025): 5362.

42. Deol, Poonamjot, Jane R. Evans, Joseph Dhahbi et al. "Soybean Oil Is More Obesogenic and Diabetogenic Than Coconut Oil and Fructose in Mouse: Potential Role for the Liver." *PLoS One* 10, no. 7 (2015): e0132672.

43. Schroeder, Henrik, Martin Werner, Dirk-Roelfs Meyer et al. "Low-Dose Paclitaxel-Coated Versus Uncoated Percutaneous Transluminal Balloon Angioplasty for Femoropopliteal Peripheral Artery Disease: One-Year Results of the ILLUMENATE European Randomized Clinical Trial (Randomized Trial of a Novel Paclitaxel-Coated Percutaneous Angioplasty Balloon)." *Circulation* 135, no. 23 (2017): 2227–36.

44. Yang, You, Xile Jiang, Stephen J. Pandol, Yuan-Ping Han, and Xiaofeng Zheng. "Green Plant Pigment, Chlorophyllin, Ameliorates Non-alcoholic Fatty Liver Diseases (NAFLDs) Through Modulating Gut Microbiome in Mice." *Frontiers in Physiology* 12 (2021): 739174.

45. Forster, J., R. Delcore, K. M. Payne, and E. L. Siegel. "The Role of Transjugular Intrahepatic Portosystemic Shunts in the Manage-

ment of Patients with End-Stage Liver Disease." *American Journal of Surgery* 168, no. 6 (1994): 592–96; discussion, 596–97.

46. Lee, Sung-Bum Lee, Byungwook Yoo, Chaemin Baeg et al. "A 12-Week, Randomized, Double-Blind, Placebo-Controlled Study to Evaluate the Efficacy and Safety of *Lactobacillus plantarum* LMT1-48 on Body Fat Loss." *Nutrients* 17, no. 7 (2025): 1191.

47. Aalipanah, Erfaneh, Moein Askarpour, Mohammad Hadi Eskandari et al. "Comparing the Effects of Yogurt Containing *Akkermansia muciniphilia* Postbiotic with Yogurt Containing *Lactobacillus rhamnosus* Postbiotic on Body Composition, Biochemical Indices, Appetite, and Depression Scores in Overweight or Obese Adults: A Randomized, Double-Blind, Controlled Clinical Trial." *Clinical Nutrition ESPEN* 68 (2025): 438–46.

48. Glisovic, S.J., Y. D. Pastore, V. Gagne et al. "Impact of Genetic Polymorphisms Determining Leukocyte/Neutrophil Count on Chemotherapy Toxicity." *Pharmacogenomics Journal* 18, no. 2 (2018): 270–74.

49. Bes-Rastrollo, Maira, Joan Sabaté, Enrique Gómez-Gracia, Alvaro Alonso, J. Alfredo Martínez, and Miguel Angel Martínez-González. "Nut Consumption and Weight Gain in a Mediterranean Cohort: The SUN Study." *Obesity* 15, no. 1 (2007): 107–16.

50. Zarbo, Allison, Kedar Inamdar, and Ben J. Friedman. "Tender Nodules on the Extremities: Challenge." *American Journal of Dermatopathology* 42, no. 11 (2020): e149–50.

51. El-Maraghy, Shohda A., Ola Adel, Naglaa Zayod, Ayman Yosry, Saeed M. El-Nahaas, and Abdullah A. Gibriel. "Circulatory miRNA-484, 524, 615 and 628 Expression Profiling in HCV Mediated HCC Among Egyptian Patients; Implications for Diagnosis and Staging of Hepatic Cirrhosis and Fibrosis." *Journal of Advanced Research* 22 (2020): 57–66.

52. Parkin, William M., and Marija Drndić. "Signal and Noise in FET-Nanopore Devices." *ACS Sensors* 3, no. 2 (2018): 313–19.

53. Rautiainen, Susanne, Lu Wang, I-Min Lee, JoAnn E. Manson, Julie E. Buring, and Howard D. Sesso. "Dairy Consumption in Association with Weight Change and Risk of Becoming Overweight or Obese in Middle-Aged and Older Women: A Prospective Cohort Study." *American Journal of Clinical Nutrition* 103, no. 4 (2016): 979–88.

54. White, Mark J., Hongjun He, Renee M. Penoske, Sally S. Twining, and Thomas C. Zahrt. "PepD participates in the Mycobacterial Stress Response Mediated Through MprAB and SigE." *Journal of Bacteriology* 192, no. 6 (2010): 1498–510.

55. Alexdottir, Marta S., Martin Pehrsson, Viktor Domislovic et al. "Neutrophil-Mediated Type IV Collagen Degradation Is Elevated in Patients with Mild Endoscopic Ulcerative Colitis Reflecting Early Mucosal Destruction." *Scientific Reports* 14, no. 1 (2024): 1641.

56. Kim, Soriul, Ki Yeol Lee, Nan Hee Kim et al. "Relationship of Obstructive Sleep Apnoea Severity and Subclinical Systemic Atherosclerosis." *European Respiratory Journal* 55, no. 2 (2020): 1900959.

57. Abd-Elmonsef Mahmoud, Ghada, and Shymaa Ryhan Bashandy. "Nitrogen, Amino Acids, and Carbon as Control Factors of Riboflavin Production by Novosphingobium panipatense-SR3 (MT002778)." *Current Microbiology* 78, no. 4 (2021): 1577–89.

58. Wastyk, Hannah C., Gabriela K. Fragiadakis, Dalia Perelman et al. "Gut-Microbiota-Targeted Diets Modulate Human Immune Status." *Cell* 184, no. 16 (2021): 4137–53.

59. Al-Zoubi, Julie. "82 Percent of Avocado Oil Adulterated, Mislabeled or Poor Quality, Study Finds." Olive Oil Times, June 22, 2020, https://www.oliveoiltimes.com/business/82-percent-of-avocado-oil-adulterated-mislabeled-or-poor-quality-study-finds/83502.

60. Depa, Keshava R. "Food Fraud in Olive Oils." *Journal of Oil Petroleum Natural Gas Reserves*, December 31, 2024.

61. Qin, Pei, Ming Zhang, Minghui Han et al. "Fried-food Consumption and Risk of Cardiovascular Disease and All-Cause Mortality: A Meta-Analysis of Observational Studies." *Heart* 107, no. 19 (2021): 1567–75.

62. Calvanese, Chiara Maria, Francesco Villani, Danilo Ercolini, and Francesca De Filippis. "Postbiotics Versus Probiotics: Possible New Allies for Human Health." *Food Research International* 217 (2025): 116869.

Chapter 6: GLP-1 and Akker's Secret Weapon

1. Spreckley, Eleanor, and Kevin Graeme Murphy. "The L-Cell in Nutritional Sensing and the Regulation of Appetite." *Frontiers in Nutrition* 2 (2015): 23.

2. Rigottier-Gois, Lionel. "Dysbiosis in Inflammatory Bowel Diseases: The Oxygen Hypothesis." *ISME Journal* 7, no. 7 (2013): 1256–61.

3. Psichas, Arianna, Leslie L. Glass, Stephen J. Sharp, Frank Reimann, and Fiona M. Gribble. "Galanin Inhibits GLP-1 and GIP Secretion Via the GAL1 Receptor in Enteroendocrine L and K Cells." *British Journal of Pharmacology* 173, no. 5 (2016): 888–98.

4. Huang, Yanling, Haocong Mo, Jie Yang et al. "Mechano-Regulation of GLP-1 Production by Piezo1 in Intestinal L Cells." *eLife*, October 14, 2024, https://elifesciences.org/reviewed-preprints/97854.

5. Cho, Young Min, Yukihiro Fujita, and Timothy J. Kieffer. "Glucagon-Like Peptide-1: Glucose Homeostasis and Beyond." *Annual Review of Physiology* 76 (2014): 535–59.

6. Moran, Timothy H., Ulrika Smedh, Kimberly P. Kinzig, Karen A. Scott, Susan Knipp, and Ellen E. Ladenheim. "Peptide YY(3-36) Inhibits Gastric Emptying and Produces Acute Reductions in Food Intake in Rhesus Monkeys." *American Journal of Physiology: Regulatory, Integrative, and Comparative Physiology* 288, no. 2 (2005): R384–388.

7. Chakhtoura, Marlene, Rachelle Haber, Malak Ghezzawi, Caline Rhayem, Raya Tcheroyan, and Christos S. Mantzoros. "Pharmacotherapy of Obesity: An Update on the Available Medications and Drugs Under Investigation." *EClinical Medicine* 58 (2023): 101882.

8. De Vos, Willem M., Herbert Tilg, Matthias Van Hul, and Patrice D. Cani. "Gut Microbiome and Health: Mechanistic Insights." *Gut* 71, no. 5 (2022): 1020–32.

9. Crooks, Benjamin, Nikoleta S. Stamataki, and John T. McLaughlin. "Appetite, the Enteroendocrine System, Gastrointestinal Disease and Obesity." *Proceedings of the Nutrition Society* 80, no. 1 (2021): 50–58.

10. Chambers, Edward S., Alexander Viardot, Arianna Psichas et al. "Effects of Targeted Delivery of Propionate to the Human Colon on Appetite Regulation, Body Weight Maintenance and Adiposity in Overweight Adults." *Gut* 64, no. 11 (2015): 1744–54.

11. You, Jie, Wu Liu, Yuxiong Huange et al. "*Akkermansia muciniphila* PROBIO Ameliorates Overweight Via Gut Microbiota Modulation: A Randomized Controlled Trial." *Food Science and Human Wellness*, June 12, 2025, https://www.sciopen.com/article/10.26599/FSHW.2025.9250659

12. Danowitz, Melinda, and Diva D. De Leon. "The Role of GLP-1 Signaling in Hypoglycemia Due to Hyperinsulinism." *Frontiers in Endocrinology* 13 (2022): 863184.

13. Drucker, Daniel J. "Mechanisms of Action and Therapeutic Application of Glucagon-like Peptide-1." *Cell Metabolism* 27, no. 4 (2018): 740–56.

14. Christiansen, Charlotte Bayer, Maria Buur Nordskov Gabe, Berit Svendsen, Lars Ove Dragsted, Mette Marie Rosenkilde, and Jens Juul Holst. "The Impact of Short-Chain Fatty Acids on GLP-1 and PYY Secretion from the Isolated Perfused Rat Colon." *American Journal of Physiology: Gastrointestinal and Liver Physiology* 315, no. 1 (2018): G53–65.

15. Maurer, Alan H., Michael Camilleri, Kevin Donohoe et al. "The SNMMI and EANM Practice Guideline for Small-Bowel and Colon Transit 1.0." *Journal of Nuclear Medicine* 54, no. 11 (2013): 2004–13.

16. Cai, Cindy X., Michelle Hribar, Sally Baxter et al. "Semaglutide and Nonarteritic Anterior Ischemic Optic Neuropathy." *JAMA Ophthalmology* 143, no. 4 (2025): 304–14.

17. Yun, Sumi, Sukmook Lee, Ho-Young Lee, Hyeon Jeong Oh, Yoonjin Kwak, and Hye Seung Lee. "Clinicopathologic and Prognostic Association of GRP94 Expression in Colorectal Cancer with Synchronous and Metachronous Metastases." *International Journal of Molecular Science* 22, no. 13 (2021): 7042.

18. Du, Liqing, Zhaozhou Zhang, Lixiang Zhai et al. "Altered Gut Microbiota-Host Bile Acid Metabolism in IBS-D Patients with Liver Depression and Spleen Deficiency Pattern." *Chinese Medicine* 18, no. 1 (2023): 87.

19. Thomas, Charles, Antimo Gioiello, Lilia Noriega et al. "TGR5-Mediated Bile Acid Sensing Controls Glucose Homeostasis." *Cell Metabolism* 10, no. 3 (2009): 167–77.

20. Cani, Patrice D., and Claude Knauf. "A Newly Identified Protein from *Akkermansia muciniphila* Stimulates GLP-1 Secretion." *Cell Metabolism* 33, no. 6 (2021): 1073–75.

21. Kang, Eun-Jung, Jae-Hoon Kim, Young Eun Kim et al. "The Secreted Protein Amuc_1409 from *Akkermansia muciniphila* Improves Gut Health Through Intestinal Stem Cell Regulation." *Nature Communications* 15, no. 1 (2024): 2983.

22. Chong, Deborah L. W., Carine Rebeyrol, Ricardo J. José et al. "ICAM-1 and ICAM-2 Are Differentially Expressed and Up-Regulated on Inflamed Pulmonary Epithelium, but Neither ICAM-2 nor LFA-1: ICAM-1 Are Required for Neutrophil Migration Into the Airways In Vivo." *Frontiers in Immunology* 12 (2021): 691957.

23. Yoon, Hyo Shin, Chung Hwan Cho, Myeong Sik Yun et al. "*Akkermansia muciniphila* Secretes a Glucagon-Like Peptide-1-Inducing Protein That Improves Glucose Homeostasis and Ameliorates Metabolic Disease in Mice." *Nature Microbiology* 6, no. 5 (2021): 563–73.

24. Salminen, Seppo, Maria Carmen Collado, Akihito Endo et al. "The International Scientific Association of Probiotics and Prebiotics (ISAPP) Consensus Statement on the Definition and Scope of Postbiotics." Nature Reviews: Gastroenterology and Hepatology 18, no. 9 (2021): 649–67.

25. Nazarinejad, Zahra, Roghayeh Molani-Gol, Leila Roozbeh Nasiraie, and Vahideh Ebrahimzadeh-Attari. "Postbiotics as a Novel Intervention for Obesity Management and Improving Metabolic Parameters: A Systematic Review and Meta-Analysis of Animal Studies." *Journal of Translational Medicine* 23, no. 1 (2025): 913.

26. Wilding, John P. H., Rachel L. Batterham, Salvatore Calanna et al. "Once-Weekly Semaglutide in Adults with Overweight or Obesity." *New England Journal of Medicine* 384, no. 11 (2021): 989–1002.

27. Hijová, Emília, Izabela Bertková, and Jana Štofilová. "Incorporating Postbiotics into Intervention for Managing Obesity." *International Journal of Molecular Sciences* 26, no. 11 (2025): 5362.

28. Alamos, Simon, Armando Reimer, Krishna K. Niyogi, and Hernan G. Garcia. "Quantitative Imaging of RNA Polymerase II Activity in Plants Reveals the Single-Cell Basis of Tissue-Wide Transcriptional Dynamics." *Nature Plants* 7, no. 8 (2021): 1037–49.

29. Bushi, Ganesh, Mahalaqua Nazli Khatib, Shivam Rohilla et al. "Association of GLP-1 Receptor Agonists with Risk of Suicidal Ideation and Behaviour: A Systematic Review and Meta-analysis." *Diabetes Metabolism Research and Reviews* 41, no. 2 (2025): e70037.

30. Depommier, Clara, Amandine Everard, Céline Druart et al. "Supplementation with *Akkermansia muciniphila* in Overweight and Obese Human Volunteers: A Proof-of-Concept Exploratory Study." *Nature Medicine* 25, no. 7 (2019): 1096–103.

31. Qu, Linkai, Jiaxuan He, Ting Xu et al. "Therapeutic Effects of Pasteurized *Akkermansia muciniphila* on Metabolic and Behavioral Dysregulation in a Zebrafish Model of Type 2 Diabetes Mellitus Comorbid with Depression." *Journal of Functional Foods* 129 (2025): 106848.

32. Everard, Amandine, Clara Belzer, Lucie Geurts et al. "Cross-Talk Between *Akkermansia muciniphila* and Intestinal Epithelium Controls Diet-Induced Obesity." *Proceedings of the National Academy of Sciences of the United States of America* 110, no. 22 (2013): 9066–71.

33. Gao, Fangfang, Canyu Cheng, Runwei Li, Zongcun Chen, Ke Tang, and Guankui Du. "The Role of *Akkermansia muciniphila* in Maintaining Health: A Bibliometric Study." *Frontiers in Medicine* 12 (2025), https://www.frontiersin.org/journals/medicine/articles/10.3389/fmed.2025.1484656/full

34. Hagi, Tatsuro, Sharon Y. Geerlings, Bart Nijsse, and Clara Belzer. "The Effect of Bile Acids on the Growth and Global Gene Expression Profiles in *Akkermansia muciniphila*." *Applied Microbiology and Biotechnology* 104, no. 24 (2020): 10641–53.

35. Khalili, Leila, Gwoncheol Park, Ravinder Nagpal, and Gloria Salazar. "The Role of *Akkermansia muciniphila* on Improving Gut and Metabolic Health Modulation: A Meta-Analysis of Preclinical Mouse Model Studies." *Microorganisms* 12, no. 8 (2024): 1627.

36. Zhang, Yifei, Ruixin Liu, Yufei Chen et al. "*Akkermansia muciniphila* Supplementation in Patients with Overweight/Obese Type 2 Diabetes: Efficacy Depends On Its Baseline Levels in the Gut." *Cell Metabolism* 37, no. 3 (2025): 592–605.

37. "Commission Implementing Regulation (EU) 2022/168 of February 8, 2022, Authorising the Placing on the Market of Pasteurised *Akkermansia muciniphila* as a Novel Food Under Regulation (EU) 2015/2283 of the European Parliament and of the Council and amending Commission Implementing Regulation," EUR-Lex. https://eur-lex.europa.eu/eli/reg_impl/2022/168/oj/eng.

38. Fillon, Alicia, Nicole Fearnbach, Stéphanie Vieira et al. "Changes in Sedentary Time and Implicit Preference for Sedentary Behaviors in Response to a One-Month Educational Intervention in Primary School Children: Results from the Globe Trotter Pilot Cluster-Randomized Study." *International Journal of Environmental Research and Public Health* 20, no. 2 (2023): 1089.

39. Smedegaard, Stine, Ulla Kampmann, Per G. Ovesen, Henrik Støvring, and Nikolaj Rittig. "Whey Protein Premeal Lowers Postprandial Glucose Concentrations in Adults Compared with Water—The Effect of Timing, Dose, and Metabolic Status: A Systematic Review and Meta-analysis." *American Journal of Clinical Nutrition* 118, no. 2 (2023): 391–405.

Chapter 7: How Dead Probiotics Help You Lose Weight

1. Ji, Jing, Weilin Jin, Shuang-Jiang Liu, Zuoyi Jiao, and Xiangkai Li. "Probiotics, Prebiotics, and Postbiotics in Health and Disease." *MedComm* 4, no. 6 (2023): e420.

2. Salminen, Seppo, Maria Carmen Collado, Akihito Endo et al. "The International Scientific Association of Probiotics and Prebiotics (ISAPP) Consensus Statement on the Definition and Scope of Postbiotics." *Nature Reviews Gastroenterology & Hepatology* 18, no. 9 (2021): 649–67.

3. Hijová, Emília, Izabela Bertková, and Jana Štofilová. "Incorporating Postbiotics into Intervention for Managing Obesity." *International Journal of Molecular Sciences* 26, no. 11 (2025): 5362.

4. Ma, Linxi, Huaijun Tu, and Tingtao Chen. "Postbiotics in Human Health: A Narrative Review," *Nutrients* 15, no. 2 (2023): 291.

5. Yilmaz, Yusuf. "Postbiotics as Antiinflammatory and Immune-Modulating Bioactive Compounds in Metabolic Dysfunction-Associated Steatotic Liver Disease." *Molecular Nutrition and Food Research* 68, no. 23 (2024): 2400754.

6. Depommier, Clara, Amandine Everard, Céline Druart et al. "Supplementation with *Akkermansia muciniphila* in Overweight and Obese Human Volunteers: A Proof-of-Concept Exploratory Study." *Nature Medicine* 25, no. 7 (2019): 1096–103.

7. Calvanese, Chiara Maria, Francesco Villani, Danilo Ercolini, and Francesca De Filippis. "Postbiotics Versus Probiotics: Possible New Allies for Human Health." *Food Research International* 217 (2025): 116869. doi:10.1016/j.foodres.2025.116869.

8. Prajapati, Nidhi, Jinil Patel, Sachidanand Singh et al. "Postbiotic Production: Harnessing the Power of Microbial Metabolites for Health Applications." *Frontiers in Microbiology* 14 (2023): 1306192.

9. Merenstein, Daniel, Bruno Pot, Gregory Leyer et al. "Emerging Issues in Probiotic Safety: 2023 Perspectives." *Gut Microbes* 15, no. 1 (2023): 2185034.

10. Vinderola, Gabriel, Céline Druart, Luis Gosálbez, Seppo Salminen, Nina Vinot, and Sarah Lebeer. "Postbiotics in the Medical Field under the Perspective of the ISAPP Definition: Scientific, Regulatory, and Marketing Considerations." *Frontiers in Pharmacology* 14 (2023): 1239745.

11. Vinderola, Gabriel, Mary Ellen Sanders, and Seppo Salminen. "The Concept of Postbiotics." *Foods* 11, no. 8 (2022): 1077.

12. Niu, Huifang, Minfeng Zhou, Daniel Zogona et al. "*Akkermansia muciniphila*: A Potential Candidate for Ameliorating Metabolic Diseases." *Frontiers in Immunology* 15 (2024): 1370658.

13. Pellegrino, Antonio, Gaetano Coppola, Francesco Santopaolo, Antonio Gasbarrini, and Francesca Romana Ponziani. "Role of *Akkermansia* in Human Diseases: From Causation to Therapeutic Properties." *Nutrients* 15, no. 8 (2023): 1815.

14. Plovier, Hubert, Amandine Everard, Céline Druart et al. "A Purified Membrane Protein from *Akkermansia muciniphila* or the Pasteurized Bacterium Improves Metabolism in Obese and Diabetic Mice." *Nature Medicine* 23, no. 1 (2017): 107–13.

15. Schulz, Eilien, Anna Karagianni, Marcus Koch, and Gregor Fuhrmann. "Hot EVs—How Temperature Affects Extracellular Vesicles." *European Journal of Pharmaceutics and Biopharmaceutics* 146 (2020): 55–63.

16. Yoon, Hyo Shin, Chung Hwan Cho, Myeong Sik Yun et al. "*Akkermansia muciniphila* Secretes a Glucagon-Like Peptide-1–Inducing Protein That Improves Glucose Homeostasis and Ameliorates Metabolic Disease in Mice." *Nature Microbiology* 6, no. 5 (2021): 563–73.

17. Jan, Tawseefa, Rajeshwari Negi, Babita Sharma et al. "Next Generation Probiotics for Human Health: An Emerging Perspective." *Heliyon* 10, no. 16 (2024): e35980.

18. Chen, Ruochan, Ju Zou, Jiawang Chen, Xiao Zhong, Rui Kang, and Daolin Tang. "Pattern Recognition Receptors: Function, Regulation and Therapeutic Potential." *Signal Transduction and Targeted Therapy* 10, no. 1 (2025): 216.

19. Cheng, Rongrong, Wenjuan Xu, Junchao Wang, Zhengquan Tang, and Min Zhang. "The Outer Membrane Protein Amuc_1100 of

Akkermansia muciniphila Alleviates the Depression-Like Behavior of Depressed Mice Induced by Chronic Stress." *Biochemical and Biophysical Research Communications* 566 (2021): 170–76.

20. Cheng, Rongrong, Haiyan Zhu, Yan Sun, Tianrong Hang, and Min Zhang. "The Modified Outer Membrane Protein Amuc_1100 of *Akkermansia muciniphila* Improves Chronic Stress-Induced Anxiety and Depression-Like Behavior in Mice." *Food and Function* 13, no. 20 (2022): 10748–58.

21. Trefts, Elijah, and Reuben J. Shaw. "AMPK: Restoring Metabolic Homeostasis over Space and Time." *Molecular Cell* 81, no. 18 (2021): 3677–90.

22. Spaulding, Hannah R., and Zhen Yan. "AMPK and the Adaptation to Exercise." *Annual Review of Physiology* 84 (2022): 209–27.

23. Melo-Marques, Inês, Sandra Morais Cardoso, and Nuno Empadinhas. "Bacterial Extracellular Vesicles at the Interface of Gut Microbiota and Immunity." *Gut Microbes* 16, no. 1 (2024): 2396494.

24. Noori, Pegah, Fattah Sotoodehnejadnematalahi, Pooneh Rahimi, and Seyed Davar Siadat. "*Akkermansia muciniphila* and Its Extracellular Vesicles Affect Endocannabinoid System in In Vitro Model." *Digestion* 106, no. 4 (2025): 338–48.

25. Wu, Qiming, Juntao Kan, Caili Fu et al. "Insights into the Unique Roles of Extracellular Vesicles for Gut Health Modulation: Mechanisms, Challenges, and Perspectives." *Current Research in Microbial Sciences* 7 (2024): 100301.

26. Sun, Desen, Pan Chen, Yang Xi, and Jinghao Sheng. "From Trash to Treasure: The Role of Bacterial Extracellular Vesicles in Gut Health and Disease." *Frontiers in Immunology* 14 (2023): 1274295.

27. Mottawea, Walid, Basit Yousuf, Salma Sultan et al. "Multi-Level Analysis of Gut Microbiome Extracellular Vesicles–Host Interaction Reveals a Connection to Gut–Brain Axis Signaling." *Microbiology Spectrum* 13, no. 2 (2025): e0136824.

28. Wang, Ling-Yun, Li-Hong He, Li-Jun Xu, and Shi-Bo Li. "Short-Chain Fatty Acids: Bridges Between Diet, Gut Microbiota, and Health." *Journal of Gastroenterology and Hepatology* 39, no. 9 (2024): 1728–36.

29. Tan, Jian Kai, Laurence Macia, and Charles R. Mackay. "Dietary Fiber and SCFAs in the Regulation of Mucosal Immunity." *Journal of Allergy and Clinical Immunology* 151, no. 2 (2023): 361–70.

30. Li, Wenweiran, Hui Chen, and Jianguo Tang. "Interplay Between Bile Acids and Intestinal Microbiota: Regulatory Mechanisms and Therapeutic Potential for Infections." *Pathogens* 13, no. 8 (2024): 702.

31. Luz, Anna Beatriz Santana, Amanda Fernandes de Medeiros, Gidyenne Christine Bandeira Silva de Medeiros, Grasiela Piuvezam, Thaís Souza Passos, and Ana Heloneida de Araújo Morais. "Experimental Protocols Used to Mimic Gastrointestinal Protein Digestion: A Systematic Review." *Nutrients* 16, no. 15 (2024): 2398.

32. Yang, Mengxiao, Zhi Yang, David W. Everett, Elliot Paul Gilbert, Harjinder Singh, and Aiqian Ye. "Digestion of Food Proteins: The Role of Pepsin." *Critical Reviews in Food Science and Nutrition* (2025): 1–22.

33. Chai, Li-Na, Hua Wu, Xue-Jiao Wang, Li-Juan He, and Chun-Feng Guo. "The Mechanism of Antimicrobial Activity of Conjugated Bile Acids Against Lactic Acid Bacilli." *Microorganisms* 11, no. 7 (2023): 1823.

34. Rao, Sameer, and Madhusudan Grover. "Intestinal Proteases." *Current Opinion in Gastroenterology* 39, no. 6 (2023): 472–78.

35. Baral, Kshitis Chandra, and Ki Young Choi. "Barriers and Strategies for Oral Peptide and Protein Therapeutics Delivery: Update on Clinical Advances." *Pharmaceutics* 17, no. 4 (2025): 397.

36. Chathuranga, Kiramage, Yeseul Shin, Md Bashir Uddin et al. "The Novel Immunobiotic *Clostridium butyricum* S-45-5 Displays Broad-Spectrum Antiviral Activity In Vitro and In Vivo by Inducing Immune Modulation." *Frontiers in Immunology* 14 (2023): 1242183.

37. Sun, Yilan, Xiaowei Xu, Qinhua Zhang et al. "Review of Konjac Glucomannan Structure, Properties, Gelation Mechanism, and Application in Medical Biology." *Polymers* 15, no. 8 (2023): 1852.

38. Wang, Chuang, Zhenzhao Guo, Jialuo Liang et al. "An Oral Delivery Vehicle Based on Konjac Glucomannan Acetate Targeting the Colon for Inflammatory Bowel Disease Therapy." *Frontiers in Bioengineering and Biotechnology* 10 (2022): 1025155.

39. Tan, Xiang, Botao Wang, Xu Zhou, Cuiping Liu, Chen Wang, and Junying Bai. "Fecal Fermentation Behaviors of Konjac Glucomannan and Its Impacts on Human Gut Microbiota." *Food Chemistry: X* 23 (2024): 101610.

40. Fang, Yimeng, Jiahui Ma, Pengyu Lei et al. "Konjac Glucomannan: An Emerging Specialty Medical Food to Aid in the Treatment of Type 2 Diabetes Mellitus." *Foods* 12, no. 2 (2023): 363.

41. Ibrahim, Ibrahim M. "Advances in Polysaccharide-Based Oral Colon-Targeted Delivery Systems: The Journey So Far and the Road Ahead." *Cureus* 15, no. 1 (2023): e33636.

42. Brodkorb, André, Lotti Egger, Marie Alminger et al. "INFOGEST Static In Vitro Simulation of Gastrointestinal Food Digestion." *Nature Protocols* 14, no. 4 (2019): 991–1014.

43. Rasera, Gabriela Boscariol, Adriano Costa de Camargo, and Ruann Janser Soares de Castro. "Bioaccessibility of Phenolic Compounds Using the Standardized INFOGEST Protocol: A Narrative Review." *Comprehensive Reviews in Food Science and Food Safety* 22, no. 1 (2023): 260–86.

44. Reboredo-Rodríguez, P., L. Olmo-García, M. Figueiredo-González, C. González-Barreiro, A. Carrasco-Pancorbo, and B. Cancho-Grande. "Application of the INFOGEST Standardized Method to Assess the Digestive Stability and Bioaccessibility of Phenolic Compounds from Galician Extra-Virgin Olive Oil." *Journal of Agricultural and Food Chemistry* 69, no. 39 (2021): 11592–605.

45. Phùng, Thị-Thanh-Trúc, Massimiliano Gerometta, Julie Chanut et al. "Comprehensive Approach to the Protection and Controlled Release of Extremely Oxygen-Sensitive Probiotics Using Edible Polysaccharide-Based Coatings." *International Journal of Biological Macromolecules* 218 (2022): 706–19.

46. Marcial-Coba, Martín Sebastián, Tomasz Cieplak, Thiago Barbosa Cahú, Andreas Blennow, Susanne Knøchel, and Dennis Sandris Nielsen. "Viability of Microencapsulated *Akkermansia muciniphila* and *Lactobacillus plantarum* During Freeze-Drying, Storage and In Vitro Simulated Upper Gastrointestinal Tract Passage." *Food & Function* 9, no. 11 (2018): 5868–79.

47. Khan, Muhammad Tanweer, Chinmay Dwibedi, Daniel Sundh et al. "Synergy and Oxygen Adaptation for Development of Next-Generation Probiotics." *Nature* 620, no. 7973 (2023): 381–85.

48. Lu, Zheng, and James A. Imlay. "When Anaerobes Encounter Oxygen: Mechanisms of Oxygen Toxicity, Tolerance and Defence." *Nature Reviews Microbiology* 19, no. 12 (2021): 774–85.

49. Sielatycka, Katarzyna, Joanna Śliwa-Dominiak, Martyna Radaczyńska et al. "Dynamics of Active Fluorescent Units (AFU) and

Water Activity (aw) Changes in Probiotic Products—Pilot Study." *Foods* 12, no. 21 (2023): 4018.

50. Wendel, Ulrika. "Assessing Viability and Stress Tolerance of Probiotics—A Review." *Frontiers in Microbiology* 12 (2021): 818468.

51. Jordal, Peter Lüttge, Marcos González Diaz, Carlotta Morazzoni et al. "Collaborative Cytometric Inter-Laboratory Ring Test for Probiotics Quantification." *Frontiers in Microbiology* 14 (2023): 1285075.

52. Van der Ark, Kees C. H., Avis Dwi Wahyu Nugroho, Claire Berton-Carabin et al. "Encapsulation of the Therapeutic Microbe *Akkermansia muciniphila* in a Double Emulsion Enhances Survival in Simulated Gastric Conditions." *Food Research International* 102 (2017): 372–79.

53. Rau, Sameeha, Andrew Gregg, Shelby Yaceczko, and Berkeley Limketkai. "Prebiotics and Probiotics for Gastrointestinal Disorders." *Nutrients* 16, no. 6 (2024): 778.

54. Hashimoto, Kaito, Kento Dora, Yoshino Murakami et al. "Positive Impact of a 10-Min Walk Immediately After Glucose Intake on Postprandial Glucose Levels." *Scientific Reports* 15, no. 1 (2025): 22662.

55. Hernández Espinell, José R., Verónica Toro, Xin Yao, Lian Yu, Vilmalí López-Mejías, and Torsten Stelzer. "Solvent-Mediated Polymorphic Transformations in Molten Polymers: The Account of Acetaminophen." *Molecular Pharmaceutics* 19, no. 7 (2022): 2183–90.

56. Wang, Xiaofei, Yue Qi, and Hao Zheng. "Dietary Polyphenol, Gut Microbiota, and Health Benefits." *Antioxidants* 11, no. 6 (2022): 1212.

57. Hughes, Riley L., David A. Alvarado, Kelly S. Swanson, and Hannah D. Holscher. "The Prebiotic Potential of Inulin-Type Fructans: A Systematic Review." *Advances in Nutrition* 13, no. 2 (2021): 492–529.

58. Merenstein, Daniel J., Daniel J. Tancredi, J. Philip Karl et al. "Is There Evidence to Support Probiotic Use for Healthy People?" *Advances in Nutrition* 15, no. 8 (2024): 100265.

59. Swanson, Kelly S., Glenn R. Gibson, Robert Hutkins et al. "The International Scientific Association for Probiotics and Prebiotics

(ISAPP) Consensus Statement on the Definition and Scope of Synbiotics." *Nature Reviews Gastroenterology & Hepatology* 17, no. 11 (2020): 687–701.

60. Mosca, Alexis, Ana Teresa Abreu Y. Abreu, Kok Ann Gwee et al. "The Clinical Evidence for Postbiotics as Microbial Therapeutics." *Gut Microbes* 14, no. 1 (2022): 2117508.

Chapter 8: The Fiber Paradox

1. Dell'Olio, Andrea, William T. Scott Jr., Silvia Taroncher-Ferrer, Nadia San Onofre, José Miguel Soriano, and Josep Rubert. "Tailored Impact of Dietary Fibers on Gut Microbiota: A Multi-Omics Comparison on the Lean and Obese Microbial Communities." *Microbiome* 12, no. 1 (2024): 250.

2. Lachmansingh, David Antoine, Benjamin Valderrama, Thomaz Bastiaanssen, John Cryan, Gerard Clarke, and Aonghus Lavelle. "Impact of Dietary Fiber on Gut Microbiota Composition, Function and Gut-Brain-Modules in Healthy Adults—a Systematic Review Protocol." *HRB Open Research* 6 (2024): 62.

3. Sonnenburg, Erica D., Samuel A. Smits, Mikhail Tikhonov, Steven K. Higginbottom, Ned S. Wingreen, and Justin L. Sonnenburg. "Diet-Induced Extinctions in the Gut Microbiota Compound over Generations." *Nature* 529, no. 7585 (2016): 212–15.

4. Meldrum, Oliver W., and Gleb E. Yakubov. "Journey of Dietary Fiber along the Gastrointestinal Tract: Role of Physical Interactions, Mucus, and Biochemical Transformations." *Critical Reviews in Food Science and Nutrition* 65, no. 22 (August 2024): 4264–92. https://www.tandfonline.com/doi/full/10.1080/10408398.2024.2390556.

5. Rous, Colombe, Julie Cadiou, Hiba Yazbek et al. "Temporary Dietary Fiber Depletion Prompts Rapid and Lasting Gut Microbiota Restructuring in Mice." *Microbiology Spectrum* 13, no. 3 (2025): e0151724.

6. Feng, Yiming, Qing Jin, Xuanbo Liu, Tiantian Lin, Andrea Johnson, and Haibo Huang. "Advances in Understanding Dietary Fiber: Classification, Structural Characterization, Modification, and Gut Microbiome Interactions." *Comprehensive Reviews in Food Science and Food Safety* 24, no. 1 (2025): e70092.

7. Xi, Na, Xiao Yang, Jie Liu, Hao Yue, and Ziyuan Wang. "Effects of Dietary Fiber Supplementation on Chronic Constipation in the

Elderly: A Systematic Review and Meta-Analysis of Randomized Controlled Trials." *Foods* 14, no. 13 (2025): 2315.

8. Bulsiewicz, Will. "The Importance of Dietary Fiber for Metabolic Health." *American Journal of Lifestyle Medicine* 17, no. 5 (2023): 639–48.

9. Chambers, Edward S., Alexander Viardot, Arianna Psichas et al. "Effects of Targeted Delivery of Propionate to the Human Colon on Appetite Regulation, Body Weight Maintenance and Adiposity in Overweight Adults." *Gut* 64, no. 11 (2015): 1744–54.

10. Friedman, Elliot S., Kyle Bittinger, Tatiana V. Esipova et al. "Microbes vs. Chemistry in the Origin of the Anaerobic Gut Lumen." *Proceedings of the National Academy of Sciences of the United States of America* 115, no. 16 (2018): 4170–75.

11. Moncada, Edward, Nuseybe Bulut, Shiyu Li, Timothy Johnson, Bruce Hamaker, and Lavanya Reddivari. "Dietary Fiber's Physicochemical Properties and Gut Bacterial Dysbiosis Determine Fiber Metabolism in the Gut." *Nutrients* 16, no. 15 (2024): 2446.

12. Zong, Wenjing, Elliot S. Friedman, Srinivasa Rao Allu et al. "Disruption of Intestinal Oxygen Balance in Acute Colitis Alters the Gut Microbiome." *Gut Microbes* 16, no. 1 (2024): 2361493.

13. Camilleri, Michael. "What Is the Leaky Gut? Clinical Considerations in Humans." *Current Opinion in Clinical Nutrition and Metabolic Care* 24, no. 5 (2021): 473–82.

14. Bertin, Luisa, Miriana Zanconato, Martina Crepaldi et al. "The Role of the FODMAP Diet in IBS." *Nutrients* 16, no. 3 (2024): 370.

15. Mohammad, Shireen, and Christoph Thiemermann. "Role of Metabolic Endotoxemia in Systemic Inflammation and Potential Interventions." *Frontiers in Immunology* 11 (2020): 594150.

16. Macura, Barbara, Aneta Kiecka, and Marian Szczepanik. "Intestinal Permeability Disturbances: Causes, Diseases and Therapy." *Clinical and Experimental Medicine* 24, no. 1 (2024): 232.

17. Hessler, Giuliana, Stephan Michael Portheine, Eva-Maria Gerlach et al. "PMR4-Dependent Cell Wall Depositions Are a Consequence but Not the Cause of Temperature-Induced Autoimmunity." *Journal of Experimental Botany,* September 14, 2021, erab423. doi:10.1093/jxb/erab423.

18. Goodoory, Vivek C., Mais Khasawneh, Christopher J. Black, Eamonn M. M. Quigley, Paul Moayyedi, and Alexander C. Ford.

"Efficacy of Probiotics in Irritable Bowel Syndrome: Systematic Review and Meta-Analysis." *Gastroenterology* 165, no. 5 (2023): 1206–18.

19. Aalipanah, Erfaneh, Moein Askarpour, Mohammad Hadi Eskandari et al. "Comparing the Effects of Yogurt Containing *Akkermansia muciniphila* Postbiotic with Yogurt Containing *Lactobacillus rhamnosus* Postbiotic on Body Composition, Biochemical Indices, Appetite, and Depression Scores in Overweight or Obese Adults: A Randomized, Double-Blind, Controlled Clinical Trial." *Clinical Nutrition ESPEN* 68 (2025): 438–46. doi:10.1016/j.clnesp.2025.05.045.

20. Akhlaghi, Mahsa. "The Role of Dietary Fibers in Regulating Appetite: An Overview of Mechanisms and Weight Consequences." *Critical Reviews in Food Science and Nutrition* 64, no. 10 (2024): 3139–50.

21. Giuntini, Eliana B., Flavia A. H. Sardá, and Eliane W. de Menezes. "The Effects of Soluble Dietary Fibers on Glycemic Response: An Overview and Future Perspectives." *Foods* 11, no. 23 (2022): 3934.

22. Van der Schoot, Alice, Candice Drysdale, Kevin Whelan, and Eirini Dimidi. "The Effect of Fiber Supplementation on Chronic Constipation in Adults: An Updated Systematic Review and Meta-Analysis of Randomized Controlled Trials." *American Journal of Clinical Nutrition* 116, no. 4 (2022): 953–69.

23. Kadyan, Saurabh, Aditya Sharma, Bahram H. Arjmandi, Prashant Singh, and Ravinder Nagpal. "Prebiotic Potential of Dietary Beans and Pulses and Their Resistant Starch for Aging-Associated Gut and Metabolic Health." *Nutrients* 14, no. 9 (2022): 1726.

24. Chen, Zhao, Ning Liang, Haili Zhang et al. "Resistant Starch and the Gut Microbiome: Exploring Beneficial Interactions and Dietary Impacts." *Food Chemistry: X* 21 (2024): 101118.

25. Zannini, Emanuele, Ángela Bravo Núñez, Aylin W. Sahin, and Elke K. Arendt. "Arabinoxylans as Functional Food Ingredients: A Review." *Foods* 11, no. 7 (2022): 1026.

26. Ghavami, Abed, Rahele Ziaei, Sepide Talebi et al. "Soluble Fiber Supplementation and Serum Lipid Profile: A Systematic Review and Dose-Response Meta-Analysis of Randomized Controlled Trials." *Advances in Nutrition* 14, no. 3 (2023): 465–74.

27. Cummings, John H., and Glenn T. Macfarlane. "Role of Intestinal Bacteria in Nutrient Metabolism." *JPEN: Journal of Parenteral and Enteral Nutrition* 21, no. 6 (1997): 357–65.

28. Amini, Shirin, Anahita Mansoori, and Leila Maghsumi-Norouzabad. "The Effect of Acute Consumption of Resistant Starch on Appetite in Healthy Adults: A Systematic Review and Meta-Analysis of the Controlled Clinical Trials." *Clinical Nutrition ESPEN* 41 (2021): 42–48.

29. So, Daniel, Chu K. Yao, Peter R. Gibson, and Jane G. Muir. "Evaluating Tolerability of Resistant Starch 2, Alone and in Combination with Minimally Fermented Fibre for Patients with Irritable Bowel Syndrome: A Pilot Randomised Controlled Cross-over Trial." *Journal of Nutritional Science* 11 (2022): e15.

30. Müller, Mattea, Gerben D. A. Hermes, Emanuel E. Canfora et al. "Effect of Wheat Bran Derived Prebiotic Supplementation on Gastrointestinal Transit, Gut Microbiota, and Metabolic Health: A Randomized Controlled Trial in Healthy Adults with a Slow Gut Transit." *Gut Microbes* 12, no. 1 (2020): 1704141.

31. Culp, Evan J., and Andrew L. Goodman. "Cross-Feeding in the Gut Microbiome: Ecology and Mechanisms." *Cell Host and Microbe* 31, no. 4 (2023): 485–99.

32. Chen, Hong, Wei Wang, Jeroen Degroote et al. "Arabinoxylan in Wheat Is More Responsible than Cellulose for Promoting Intestinal Barrier Function in Weaned Male Piglets." *Journal of Nutrition* 145, no. 1 (2015): 51–58.

33. Ciupei, Daria, Alexandru Colişar, Loredana Leopold, Andreea Stănilă, and Zoriţa M. Diaconeasa. "Polyphenols: From Classification to Therapeutic Potential and Bioavailability." *Foods* 13, no. 24 (2024): 4131.

34. Singh, Neeraj, and S. S. Yadav. "A Review on Health Benefits of Phenolics Derived from Dietary Spices." *Current Research in Food Science* 5 (2022): 1508–23.

35. Cheng, Hao, Dandan Zhang, Jing Wu et al. "Interactions between Gut Microbiota and Polyphenols: A Mechanistic and Metabolomic Review." *Phytomedicine* 119 (2023): 154979.

36. Rudrapal, Mithun, Shubham J. Khairnar, Johra Khan et al. "Dietary Polyphenols and Their Role in Oxidative Stress-Induced Human Diseases: Insights into Protective Effects, Antioxidant

Potentials and Mechanism(s) of Action." *Frontiers in Pharmacology* 13 (2022): 806470.

37. Gade, Anushree, and Maushmi S. Kumar. "Gut Microbial Metabolites of Dietary Polyphenols and Their Potential Role in Human Health and Diseases." *Journal of Physiology and Biochemistry* 79, no. 4 (2023): 695–718.

38. Scott, Michael B., Amy K. Styring, and James S. O. McCullagh. "Polyphenols: Bioavailability, Microbiome Interactions and Cellular Effects on Health in Humans and Animals." *Pathogens* 11, no. 7 (2022): 770.

39. Munteanu, Camelia, and Betty Schwartz. "Interactions between Dietary Antioxidants, Dietary Fiber and the Gut Microbiome: Their Putative Role in Inflammation and Cancer." *International Journal of Molecular Sciences* 25, no. 15 (2024): 8250.

40. Wang, Xiang, Yue Qi, and Hao Zheng. "Dietary Polyphenol, Gut Microbiota, and Health Benefits." *Antioxidants* 11, no. 6 (2022): 1212.

41. Bouyahya, Abdelhakim, Nasreddine El Omari, Naoufal El Hachlafi et al. "Chemical Compounds of Berry-Derived Polyphenols and Their Effects on Gut Microbiota, Inflammation, and Cancer." *Molecules* 27, no. 10 (2022): 3286.

42. Henning, Susanne M., Paula H. Summanen, Ru-Po Lee et al. "Pomegranate Ellagitannins Stimulate the Growth of *Akkermansia muciniphila* In Vivo." *Anaerobe* 43 (2017): 56–60.

43. Au, Hezekiah C. T., Yang Jing Zheng, Gia Han Le et al. "Association of Glucagon-Like Peptide-1 Receptor Agonists (GLP-1 RAs) and Neurogenesis: A Systematic Review." *Acta Neuropsychiatrica* 37 (2025): e50.

44. Anhê, Fernando F., Denis Roy, Geneviève Pilon et al. "A Polyphenol-Rich Cranberry Extract Protects from Diet-Induced Obesity, Insulin Resistance and Intestinal Inflammation in Association with Increased *Akkermansia* spp. Population in the Gut Microbiota of Mice." *Gut* 64, no. 6 (2015): 872–83.

45. Jawhara, Samir. "How Do Polyphenol-Rich Foods Prevent Oxidative Stress and Maintain Gut Health?" *Microorganisms* 12, no. 8 (2024): 1570.

46. Rana, Ananya, Mrinal Samtiya, Tejpal Dhewa, Vijendra Mishra, and Rotimi E. Aluko. "Health Benefits of Polyphenols: A

Concise Review." *Journal of Food Biochemistry* 46, no. 10 (2022): e14264.

47. Konjar, Špela, Miha Pavšič, AND Marc Veldhoen. "Regulation of Oxygen Homeostasis at the Intestinal Epithelial Barrier Site." *International Journal of Molecular Sciences* 22, no. 17 (2021): 9170.

48. Vinelli, Valentina, Paola Biscotti, Daniela Martini et al. "Effects of Dietary Fibers on Short-Chain Fatty Acids and Gut Microbiota Composition in Healthy Adults: A Systematic Review." *Nutrients* 14, no. 13 (2022): 2559.

49. Lacy, Brian E., Mark Pimentel, Darren M. Brenner et al. "ACG Clinical Guideline: Management of Irritable Bowel Syndrome." *American Journal of Gastroenterology* 116, no. 1 (2021): 17–44.

50. Rijnaarts, Iris, Nicole M. de Roos, Taojun Wang et al. "A High-Fibre Personalised Dietary Advice Given via a Web Tool Reduces Constipation Complaints in Adults." *Journal of Nutritional Science* 11 (2022): e31.

51. Morishita, Daisuke, Toshihiko Tomita, Sumire Mori et al. "Senna Versus Magnesium Oxide for the Treatment of Chronic Constipation: A Randomized, Placebo-Controlled Trial." *American Journal of Gastroenterology* 116, no. 1 (2021): 152–61.

52. Kohanmoo, Ali, Shiva Faghih, and Masoumeh Akhlaghi. "Effect of Short- and Long-Term Protein Consumption on Appetite and Appetite-Regulating Gastrointestinal Hormones: A Systematic Review and Meta-Analysis of Randomized Controlled Trials." *Physiology and Behavior* 226 (2020): 113123.

53. Lu, Kun, Tingqing Yu, Xinyi Cao et al. "Effect of Viscous Soluble Dietary Fiber on Glucose and Lipid Metabolism in Patients with Type 2 Diabetes Mellitus: A Systematic Review and Meta-Analysis on Randomized Clinical Trials." *Frontiers in Nutrition* 10 (2023): 1253312.

54. Benedicto-Toboso, M. Isabel, Andressa Freire Salviano, María L. Miguel-Berges, Isabel Rueda-De Torre, Luis A. Moreno, and Alba M. Santaliestra-Pasías. "Effect of Dietary Fiber Intake on Chronic Low-Grade Inflammation in Children and Adolescents: A Systematic Review and Meta-Analysis of Randomized Controlled Trials." *Current Developments in Nutrition* 9, no. 9 (2025): 107511.

55. Strozyk, Sylwia, Anita Rogowicz-Frontczak, Stanislaw Pilacinski, Joanna LeThanh-Blicharz, Anna Koperska, and Dorota Zozulinska-Ziolkiewicz. "Influence of Resistant Starch Resulting

from the Cooling of Rice on Postprandial Glycemia in Type 1 Diabetes." *Nutrition and Diabetes* 12, no. 1 (2022): 21.

56. Trunckle Baptista, Nathália, Robin Dessalles, Anne-Kathrin Illner et al. "Harnessing the Power of Resistant Starch: A Narrative Review of Its Health Impact and Processing Challenges." *Frontiers in Nutrition* 11 (2024): 1369950.

57. Munir, Haroon, Hamza Alam, Muhammad Tahir Nadeem, Riyadh S. Almalki, Muhammad Sajid Arshad, and Hafiz Ansar Rasul Suleria. "Green Banana Resistant Starch: A Promising Potential as Functional Ingredient against Certain Maladies." *Food Science and Nutrition* 12, no. 6 (2024): 3787–805.

58. Bhardwaj, Kanchan, Agnieszka Najda, Ruchi Sharma et al. "Fruit and Vegetable Peel-Enriched Functional Foods: Potential Avenues and Health Perspectives." *Evidence-Based Complementary and Alternative Medicine* (2022): 8543881.

59. Timm, Madeline, Lisa C. Offringa, B. Jan-Willem Van Klinken, and Joanne Slavin. "Beyond Insoluble Dietary Fiber: Bioactive Compounds in Plant Foods." *Nutrients* 15, no. 19 (2023): 4138.

60. Fernandes, Ana, Nuno Mateus, and Victor de Freitas. "Polyphenol-Dietary Fiber Conjugates from Fruits and Vegetables: Nature and Biological Fate in a Food and Nutrition Perspective." *Foods* 12, no. 5 (2023): 1052.

Chapter 9: A Two-Step Restoration Protocol

1. Neurath, Markus F., David Artis, and Christoph Becker. "The Intestinal Barrier: A Pivotal Role in Health, Inflammation, and Cancer." *Lancet: Gastroenterology and Hepatology* 10, no. 6 (2025): 573–92.

2. Xi, Menglu, Guo Hao, Qi Yao, Xuchang Duan, and Wupeng Ge. "Galactooligosaccharide Mediates NF-κB Pathway to Improve Intestinal Barrier Function and Intestinal Microbiota." *Molecules* 28, no. 22 (2023): 7611.

3. Li, Dan, Yujuan Li, Shengjie Yang, Jing Lu, Xiao Jin, and Min Wu. "Diet-Gut Microbiota-Epigenetics in Metabolic Diseases: From Mechanisms to Therapeutics." *Biomedicine and Pharmacotherapy* 153 (2022): 113290.

4. Li, Hang-Yu, Dan-Dan Zhou, Ren-You Gan et al. "Effects and Mechanisms of Probiotics, Prebiotics, Synbiotics, and Postbiot-

ics on Metabolic Diseases Targeting Gut Microbiota: A Narrative Review." *Nutrients* 13, no. 9 (2021): 3211.

5. Gibbons, Sean M., Thomas Gurry, Johanna W. Lampe et al. "Perspective: Leveraging the Gut Microbiota to Predict Personalized Responses to Dietary, Prebiotic, and Probiotic Interventions." *Advances in Nutrition* 13, no. 5 (2022): 1450–61.

6. Zheng, Yanfei, Zengliang Zhang, Ping Tang et al. "Probiotics Fortify Intestinal Barrier Function: A Systematic Review and Meta-Analysis of Randomized Trials." *Frontiers in Immunology* 14 (2023): 1143548.

7. You, Jie, Wu Liu, Yuxiong Huange et al. "*Akkermansia muciniphila* PROBIO Ameliorates Overweight Via Gut Microbiota Modulation: A Randomized Controlled Trial." *Food Science and Human Wellness*, June 12, 2025. https://www.sciopen.com/article/10.26599/FSHW.2025.9250659.

8. Cani, Patrice D., and Claude Knauf. "A Newly Identified Protein from *Akkermansia muciniphila* Stimulates GLP-1 Secretion." *Cell Metabolism* 33, no. 6 (2021): 1073–5.

9. Christie, William W., and John L. Harwood. "Oxidation of Polyunsaturated Fatty Acids to Produce Lipid Mediators." *Essays in Biochemistry* 64, no. 3 (2020): 401–21.

10. Deol, Poonamjot, Paul Ruegger, Geoffrey D. Logan et al. "Diet High in Linoleic Acid Dysregulates the intestinal Endocannabinoid System and increases Susceptibility to Colitis in Mice." *Gut Microbes* 15, no. 1 (2023): 2229945.

11. Plovier, Hubert, Amandine Everard, Céline Druart et al. "A Purified Membrane Protein from *Akkermansia muciniphila* or the Pasteurized Bacterium Improves Metabolism in Obese and Diabetic Mice." *Nature Medicine* 23, no. 1 (2017): 107–13.

12. Salminen, Seppo, Maria Carmen Collado, Akihito Endo et al. "The International Scientific Association of Probiotics and Prebiotics (ISAPP) Consensus Statement on the Definition and Scope of Postbiotics." *Nature Reviews: Gastroenterology and Hepatology* 18, no. 9 (2021): 649–67.

13. Turck, Dominique, Torsten Bohn, Jacqueline Castenmiller et al. "Safety of Pasteurised *Akkermansia muciniphila* as a Novel Food Pursuant to Regulation (EU) 2015/2283." *EFSA Journal* 19, no. 9 (2021): e06780.

14. Qu, Linkai, Jiaxuan He, Ting Xu et al. "Therapeutic Effects of Pasteurized *Akkermansia muciniphila* on Metabolic and Behavioral Dysregulation in a Zebrafish Model of type 2 Diabetes Mellitus Comorbid with Depression." *Journal of Funct Foods* 129 (2025): 106848.

15. Bakhtiary, Mahsa, Mojgan Morvaridzadeh, Shahram Agah et al. "Effect of Probiotic, Prebiotic, and Synbiotic Supplementation on Cardiometabolic and Oxidative Stress Parameters in Patients With Chronic Kidney Disease: A Systematic Review and Meta-analysis." *Clinical Therapeutics* 43, no. 3 (2021): e71–96.

16. Gao, Fangfang, Canyu Cheng, Runwei Li, Zongcun Chen, Ke Tang, and Guankui Du. "The Role of *Akkermansia muciniphila* in Maintaining Health: A Bibliometric Study." *Frontiers in Medicine* 12 (2025), https://www.frontiersin.org/journals/medicine/articles/10.3389/fmed.2025.1484656/full.

17. Zmora, Niv, Gili Zilberman-Schapira, Jotham Suez et al. "Personalized Gut Mucosal Colonization Resistance to Empiric Probiotics Is Associated with Unique Host and Microbiome Features." *Cell* 174, no. 6 (2018): 1388–1405.

18. Yang, Yi-Meng, Meng-Yue Zhang, Ying-Ying Wu, Lu Zhang, and Yi-Xuan Zhang. "Survival and Morphological Changes of *Clostridium butyricum* Spores Co-Exposed to Antibiotics and Simulated Gastrointestinal Fluids: Implications for Antibiotic Stewardship." *Microorganisms* 13, no, 6 (2025): 1347.

19. Pei, Zhangming, Yufei Liu, Zhi Yi et al. "Diversity within the Species *Clostridium butyricum*: Pan-Genome, Phylogeny, Prophage, Carbohydrate Utilization, and Antibiotic Resistance." *Journal of Applied Microbiology* 134, no. 7 (2023): lxad127.

20. Xie, Yajuan, Luoning Gou, Miaomiao Peng, Juan Zheng, and Lulu Chen. "Effects of Soluble Fiber Supplementation on Glycemic Control in Adults with Type 2 Diabetes Mellitus: A Systematic Review and Meta-Analysis of Randomized Controlled Trials." *Clinical Nutrition* 40, no. 4 (2021): 1800–10.

21. Xu, Renfan, Yang Bai, Ke Yang, and Guangzhi Chen. "Effects of Green Tea Consumption on Glycemic Control: A Systematic Review and Meta-Analysis of Randomized Controlled Trials." *Nutrition and Metabolism* 17 (2020): 56.

22. Thomson, Catriona, Ada L. Garcia, and Christine A. Edwards. "Interactions Between Dietary Fibre and the Gut Microbiota." *Proceedings of the Nutrition Society* (2021): 1–11.

23. Bush, Jason R., Joshua Baisley, Scott V. Harding, and Michelle J. Alfa. "Consumption of Solnul™ Resistant Potato Starch Produces a Prebiotic Effect in a Randomized, Placebo-Controlled Clinical Trial." *Nutrients* 15, no. 7 (2023): 1582.

24. Strozyk, Sylwia, Anita Rogowicz-Frontczak, Stanislaw Pilacinski, Joanna LeThanh-Blicharz, Anna Koperska, and Dorota Zozulinska-Ziolkiewicz. "Influence of Resistant Starch Resulting from the Cooling of Rice on Postprandial Glycemia in type 1 Diabetes." Nutrition and Diabetes 12, no. 1 (2022): 21.

25. Patel, Michele L., Lindsay N. Wakayama, and Gary G. Bennett. "Self-Monitoring via Digital Health in Weight Loss Interventions: A Systematic Review Among Adults with Overweight or Obesity." *Obesity* 29, no. 3 (2021): 478–99.

26. Mouchti, Sofia, Josefina Orliacq, Gillian Reeves, and Zhengming Chen. "Assessment of Correlation Between Conventional Anthropometric and Imaging-Derived Measures of Body Fat Composition: A Systematic Literature Review and Meta-Analysis of Observational Studies." *BMC Medical Imaging* 23, no. 1 (2023): 127.

27. Ross, Robert, Ian J. Neeland, Shizuya Yamashita et al. "Waist Circumference as a Vital Sign in Clinical Practice: A Consensus Statement from the IAS and ICCR Working Group on Visceral Obesity." *Nature Reviews: Endocrinology* 16, no. 3 (2020): 177–89.

28. Ashwell, Margaret, and Sigrid Gibson. "Waist-to-Height Ratio as an Indicator of 'Early Health Risk': Simpler and More Predictive Than Using a 'Matrix'Based on BMI and Waist Circumference." *BMJ Open* 6, no. 3 (2016): e010159.

29. Kolb, Hubert. "Obese Visceral Fat Tissue Inflammation: From Protective to Detrimental?" *BMC Medicine* 20, no. 1 (2022): 494.

30. Pasanta, Duanghathai, Khin Thandar Htun, Jie Pan et al. "Waist Circumference and BMI Are Strongly Correlated with MRI-Derived Fat Compartments in Young Adults." *Life* 11, no. 7 (2021): 643.

31. Wyatt, Patrick, Sarah E. Berry, Graham Finlayson et al. "Postprandial Glycaemic Dips Predict Appetite and Energy Intake in Healthy Individuals." *Nature Metabolism* 3, no. 4 (2021): 523–29.

32. Anguah, Katherene O-B, Majid M. Syed-Abdul, Qiong Hu et al. "Changes in Food Cravings and Eating Behavior After a Dietary Carbohydrate Restriction Intervention Trial." *Nutrients* 12, no. 1 (2019): 52.

33. Scanci da Silva Pontes, Karine, Marcella Rodrigues Guedes, Michelle Rabello da Cunha et al. "Effects of Probiotics on Body Adiposity and Cardiovascular Risk Markers in Individuals with Overweight and Obesity: A Systematic Review and Meta-Analysis of Randomized Controlled Trials." *Clinical Nutrition* 40, no. 8 (2021): 4915–31.

34. Madigan, Claire D., Henrietta E. Graham, Elizabeth Sturgiss et al. "Effectiveness of Weight Management Interventions for Adults Delivered in Primary Care: Systematic Review and Meta-Analysis of Randomised Controlled Trials." *BMJ* 2022 May 30, 2022; e069719.

35. Buller, Sophie, and Clemence Blouet. "Brain Access of Incretins and Incretin Receptor Agonists to Their Central Targets Relevant for Appetite Suppression and Weight Loss." *American Journal of Physiology: Endocrinology and Metabolism* 326, no. 4 (2024): E472–80.

36. Wilding, John P.H., Rachel L. Batterham, Salvatore Calanna et al. "Once-Weekly Semaglutide in Adults with Overweight or Obesity." *New England Journal of Medicine* 384, no. 11 (2021): 989–1002.

37. Jalleh, Ryan J., Mark P. Plummer, Chinmay S. Marathe et al. "Clinical Consequences of Delayed Gastric Emptying With GLP-1 Receptor Agonists and Tirzepatide." *Journal of Clinical Endocrinology and Metabolism* 110, no. 1 (2024): 1–15.

38. Drucker, Danile J. "Efficacy and Safety of GLP-1 Medicines for Type 2 Diabetes and Obesity." *Diabetes Care* 47, no. 11 (2024): 1873–88.

39. Antoun, Jumana, Hala Itani, Natally Alarab, and Amir Elsehmawy. "The Effectiveness of Combining Nonmobile Interventions with the Use of Smartphone Apps with Various Features for Weight Loss: Systematic Review and Meta-Analysis." *JMIR mHealth uHealth* 10, no. 4 (2022): e35479.

40. Wilding, John P. H., Rachel L. Batterham, Melanie Davies et al. "Weight Regain and Cardiometabolic Effects after Withdrawal of Semaglutide: The STEP 1 Trial Extension." Diabetes, *Obesity, and Metabolism* 24, no. 8 (2022): 1553–64.

41. Li, Wanyang, and Wei Chen. "Weight Cycling Based on Altered Immune Microenvironment as a Result of Metaflammation." *Nutrition and Metabolism* 20, no. 1 (2023): 13.

List of Figures

Figure 1, page 2: GLP-1 Drugs Suppress Appetite but with Trade-Offs

Figure 2, page 3: GLP-1 Agonist

Figure 3, page 5: *Akkermansia* in the Mucus Layer

Figure 4, page 7: Microbial SCFAs Fuel Colon Cells and Signal Metabolism and Appetite

Figure 5, page 8: Gut Gems and Nutrients

Figure 6, page 9: Small Pilot Trial

Figure 7, page 11: Oxygen Gradient from Small Intestine to Colon

Figure 8, page 13: Butyrate Fuels Colonocytes and Tightens Junctions

Figure 9, page 15: Add Fermentable Fibers When the Barrier is Ready

Figure 10, page 17: High-LA Seed Oils Cause Barrier Damage and Inflammation

Figure 11, page 18: National Data Show Parallel Trends

Figure 12, page 19: Oxidized Seed Oils Thin the Mucus Layer and Generate Toxic By-products

Figure 13, page 22: L cells Release GLP-1 and PYY *Akkermansia* Proteins

Figure 14, page 23: Postbiotics are Preparations of Inanimate Microbes/Components

Figure 15, page 25: Targeted Coatings and Oxygen-safe Packaging

Figure 16, page 28: The Probiotic Gauntlet—Acid, Bile, Enzymes, and Oxygen

Figure 17, page 29: Soluble vs. Insoluble Fiber

Figure 18, page 31: Two-Phase Gut Restoration Plan

Figure 19, page 35: Real-World GLP-1 Journey

Figure 20, page 37: Hype vs. Data

Figure 21, page 38: GLP-1 Slows Gastric Emptying

Figure 22, page 40: After Stopping Semaglutide

Figure 23, page 41: Common GI Effects

Figure 24, page 43: Gastroparesis/Ileus—Know Red-Flag Symptoms

Figure 25, page 45: Rapid Weight Loss Increases Gallstone Risk

Figure 26, page 46: Monitor for Sudden Vision Changes

Figure 27, page 48: Protect Lean Mass 15–30% of Weight Loss May be Lean Tissue

Figure 28, page 50: Pause GLP-1s Pre-Procedure to Reduce Aspiration Risk

Figure 29, page 51: Mood Signals Under Investigation; Monitor for Emotional Blunting

Figure 30, page 52: Costs, Coverage, and Counterfeit Risks

Figure 31, page 54: On-Off Use Leads to Rebound and Side-Effect Reset

Figure 32, page 55: Medication as Scaffolding: Pair with Protein, Training, and Healthy Habits

Figure 33, page 61: Iceberg Blind Spot

Figure 34, page 63: Diagram of the Ileum and Colon

Figure 35, page 64: Mucus Cross-Feeding

Figure 36, page 69: PubMed Publications About Akker Rose Steeply after 2010

Figure 37, page 72: Dietary Fiber—Inulin and FOS

Figure 38, page 76: *Akkermansia* and Gut Health

Figure 39, page 81: The Repair Loop

Figure 40, page 82: Butyrate from Fiber Fuels Colonocytes

Figure 41, page 83: Butyrate and Propionate Promote Regulatory T cells

Figure 42, page 84: Gut Gem Matrix

Figure 43, page 88: Gut Barrier Tight Junctions and the Mighty Mucus Layer

Figure 44, page 89: How Colonocytes Keep it Oxygen-Free

Figure 45, page 92: Low Fiber Drives a Reinforcing Loop of Dysbiosis and Leakiness

List of Figures

Figure 46, page 98: Timeline of US Seed-Oil Adoption

Figure 47, page 99: Lipid Peroxidation Pathway

Figure 48, page 101: Aldehyde Buildup During Repeated Frying

Figure 49, page 103: Toxic Aldehydes Injure Colonocytes

Figure 50, page 105: Fragile Fat–Derived Aldehydes Trigger a Reinforcing Loop of Colonocyte Injury

Figure 51, page 107: Overlapping Western Diet Risks Converge on Gut Dysbiosis

Figure 52, page 111: Comparison of an Ultra-Processed Meal vs. a Home-Prepared Meal

Figure 53, page 114: The Ileal Brake—L cells Concentrated in the Distal Gut Sense Nutrients

Figure 54, page 115: L Cells Sense Nutrients and Gut Gems Release GLP-1 and PYY

Figure 55, page 117: Two-Layer Mucus with *Akkermansia*

Figure 56, page 121: *Akkermansia*'s Secret Weapons

Figure 57, page 123: How GLP-1 is Released

Figure 58, page 125: Evidence Snapshot of Rodent Studies

Figure 59, page 128: Lifestyle Inputs and Gut Health

Figure 60, page 134: Human Trial with *Akkermansia*

Figure 61, page 135: Pasteurized *Akkermansia* Signals

Figure 62, page 138: Dead Cell Fragments, Extracellular Vesicles, and Metabolites

Figure 63, page 140: The Digestive Gauntlet of Stomach Acid, Bile, Enzymes, and an Oxygen-Sensitive Colon Challenge Postbiotic Survival

Figure 64, page 142: The Double Shield Capsule

Figure 65, page 143: Relative Survival of Probiotics in Simulated GI Transit

Figure 66, page 144: Comparison of CFU vs. AFU Methods for Anaerobe Viability

Figure 67, page 147: Two-Stage Roadmap of Postbiotics Repair

Figure 68, page 151: Diverse Plant Fibers Feed Overlapping Microbial Guilds Across the Colon

Figure 69, page 153: Heal the Gut Barrier First then Fiber Plays Nicer

Figure 70, page 154: Leaky Gut Barrier Damage

Figure 71, page 158: Fiber and Polyphenols Act Through Complementary Microbial Pathways

Figure 72, page 160: Fiber Fermentation Fuels Colon Cells

Figure 73, page 162: Gradual Stepwise Fiber Increase

Figure 74, page 163: Cook-Cool-Reheat Boosts Resistant Starch

Figure 75, page 164: Quick-Reference Table Summarizing Major Fiber Classes

Figure 76, page 168: Repairing the Gut Barrier Prevents Toxin Leakage

Figure 77, page 169: Twelve-Week Gut Restoration Timeline

Figure 78, page 170: Cooking Fats Spectrum Swap

Figure 79, page 173: Two-Step Probiotic Strategy

Figure 80, page 175: Plate and Pantry Map of Gut-Friendly Foods

Figure 81, page 178: Progress Chart with Sparklines for Waist-to-Height Ratio

Figure 82, page 182: Two-Step Protocol Flowchart

Index

Note: Page numbers in *italics* refer to tables and figures.

A

acetate, 5, 6–7, *7–8*, 14, 82, *83–84*, 84–85, *88*, *117*, *164*

Akkermansia muciniphila (Akker), 59–78
    benefits of, 124–26, *125*
    diet and lifestyle to support, 72–75, *72*, 126–29, *128*
    fiber paradox and, *153*, 155
    GLP-1 agonist proteins, 119–22, *121*
    GLP-1 boost by, 20–22, 113–30 (*See also* GLP-1 (glucon-like peptide-1) hormone; L cells)
    healthy gut support from, 64–67, *64*
    low-oxygen environment for, 10–12, *11*, 60–62, *61*, *63*
    overview, 4–10, *5*, *7–9*, 59–60
    pasteurized Akker, 9–10, *9*, 21, 23–24, 70–71, 75, 124–27, *125*, 132–37, *134–35*, 171, 173
    polyphenols and, 158–59, *158*
    as postbiotic, 23–24 (*See also* postbiotics)
    precautions, 75–76, *76*
    research (2004) and discovery of, 59–60, *61*
    research (2008–2015), 67–70, *69*
    research (2016–2020), 70–72
    research (2021–2024), 76–77
    restoration protocol for, 171, 172–74, *173*

Victory Checkpoint, 78
weight-loss (GLP-1) drug comparison, 21–22
A-Mansia Biotech, 24
AMP-activated protein kinase (AMPK), 137, 139
AMPs (antimicrobial peptides), 86–87, 90–91
Amuc_1100 (Akker's Key)
   gut health and, *64*, 65–66
   mechanism of action, 70–71, *135*, 136–37, *138*, *153*
   overview, 20–21, *22*, 24
   restoration protocol, 183
Amuc_1409, 119, *121*, 122
antimicrobial peptides (AMPs), 86–87, 90–91
arabinoxylan (hemicellulose), 155–57, *164*
aspiration danger with GLP-1 drugs, 49–50, *50*

B

Bifidobacteria, 32
bile duct issues, 44–45, *45*
blood sugar control, 176–77, *178*, 179. *See also* insulin sensitivity and resistance
bone density loss, with GLP-1 drugs, 47–49, *48*
butyrate
   fiber and, 12–14, *13*, 29, *29*, 155–56, 159–60, *160*, *164*
   function of, 82–85, *82–84*, 87, *88–89*, 89, *117*, 186
   overview, 5, 6–7, *7–8*, 79–80
   production of, 64, *64*, 76, 174, 183
   seed oils and, 16–17, 102–3, *103*

C

cancer, 69, 92, 108
cancer immunotherapy, 67
cathelicidins, 86–87
cholesterol levels, 9, *9*, 66–67, 107–8, *125*, 126, 134, *134*, 155
choline, 66–67

Clostridium butyricum, 141, 173–74
colon and colonocytes
    cancer, 69, 92, 108
    colon-targeted probiotic delivery, 25–27, *25*, *28*
    for gut health, 79–80, *81–82*, 85–86, 88–91, *88–89*
    overview, 12–14, *13*, 16–17
    oxygen gradient for, 10–12, *11*, 60–62, *61*, *63*, 119
    seed oils and, 101–4, *103*, *105*
consumer-friendly blueprint for GLP-1 drugs. *See* weight-loss (GLP-1) drugs
corn oil. *See* seed oils
corn syrup, 30, 106
cottonseed oil. *See* seed oils
Crisco, 96–97

D
defensins, 86–87, *89*, 90–91
diabetes, 36–37, 47, 52–53, 67–69, 179
diabetic retinopathy, 47
digestive gauntlet, 25–27, *25*, *28*, 139–45, *140*, *142–44*
drugs. *See* weight-loss (GLP-1) drugs
dysbiosis, *92*, 104, *107*

E
E. coli, 104
emotional blunting, 50–51, *51*, 180
exercise, 49, 55, *55*, 56, 127, 137, 171–72
extracellular vesicles (EVs), 132–33, *135*, 137–38, *138*

F
Faecalibacterium prausnitzii, 32, 76, 174
fasting (intermittent), *72*, 73–75, 137
fermentation cascade, 159–60, *160*, 175–76

fermented foods, 33, 59–60, 110
fiber, 150–66
    cheat sheet for, 164, *164*
    fermentation cascade, 159–60, *160*, 175–76
    fiber paradox, 30–31, 152–55, *153–54*
    fiber types, 28–30, *29*, *31*, 155–57, 164, *164*
    function of, 24
    Gut Gems and, *88*
    L cells and, 118
    overview, 12–15, *13*, 109, 150–52, *151*
    plan for introducing, 146, 161–64, *162–63*
    polyphenols and, 157–59, *158*
    reality check, 30–31
    real-world win, 165
    restoration protocol and, 174–76, *175*
    Victory Checkpoint, 165–66
fitness training, 49, 55, *55*, 56, 127, 137, 171–72
4-hydroxynonenal (4-HNE), 16–17, *17*, *19*, 99–100, 102–3
fragile fats, 56, 95, 99–101, *99*. *See also* seed oils
fructooligosaccharides (FOS), *72*, 146

G

gallstones, 44–45, *45*
gastroparesis, 42, *43*, 46
GIP (glucose-dependent insulinotropic polypeptide), 118
GLP-1 (glucon-like peptide-1) hormone
    Akker and, 133, *135*
    fiber and, 151
    function of, 83, *84*, 118
    game plan for, 127
    L cells and, *114–15*, 116–18, *117*
    natural amplification of, 126–29
    new paradigm for weight loss, 186
    overview, 1, *8*, 19–22, *22*
    release of, 119–22, *121*

weight-loss drug comparison, 122–24, *123*
GLP-1 drugs. *See* weight-loss (GLP-1) drugs
glucomannan, 141–45, *142–44*, 172
glucose-dependent insulinotropic polypeptide (GIP), 118
G-protein–coupled receptors (GPCRs), 82–83, 86, 113, 116
Gut Conquests, 78
Gut Gems. *See also* acetate; butyrate; propionate
   fiber and, 155, 156, *158*, 159–60, *160*, *164*, 175–76
   function of, *115*, *117*, 118, 128
   for gut health, 80–87, *81*, *83–84*, *88*
   overview, 5, 6–7, *7–8*, 12–14, *13*
   prebiotics for, 127
   restoration protocol, 175–76
Gut Health Checkpoint, 93–94
gut microbes, 12–15, *13*, 24. *See also Akkermansia muciniphila*; postbiotics; prebiotics; probiotics

H

hemicellulose (arabinoxylan), 155–57, *164*
HIF-1α (hypoxia-inducible factor 1-alpha), *89*, 90–91, 102–3
high-fructose corn syrup, 30, 106
high-sensitivity C-reactive protein (hs-CRP), 161–62, 177, *178*
histone deacetylase (HDAC), 80, 82
HOMA-IR, 9, 176–77
hypoxia-inducible factor 1-alpha (HIF-1α), *89*, 90–91, 102–3

I

IBD (inflammatory bowel disease), 69
ICAM-2 (intercellular adhesion molecule 2), 119–20
ileus, 42, *43*, 46
immune health
   fiber for, 14, 110, 152–55
   Gut Gems and, 7, 82–87, *83–84*, *88*
   gut microbiome and, 24, 65–67, 77, 119–20, *121*

postbiotics for, 145
immunotherapy, 67
incretin, 118
inflammation
   fiber for, 29, 156, 158–59, 175–76
   fiber paradox, 152–55, *153–54*
   Gut Gems for, 6–7, *7*, 79–80, 84–85, *84*
   gut microbiome and, 21, 24, 65–69, 75, 77, 124–26, *125*, 136, 138, *138*, 158–59, 185–87
   leaky gut and, 14–15, 30, 85–86, 91–93
   polyphenols for, 73
   restoration protocol for, 32, 167–68, *168*, 169–70, 175–77, 179–80
   seed oils and, 16–19, *17*, *19*, 100, 104, *105*, 106–7, *107*, 169–70
inflammatory bowel disease (IBD), 69
insoluble fiber, 28, *29*, 155–57, *164*
insulin sensitivity and resistance
   Akker for, 8–9, *9*, 125–26, *125*, 134, *134*
   blood sugar control, 176–77, *178*, 179
   GLP-1 boost and, 21–22
intercellular adhesion molecule 2 (ICAM-2), 119–20, *121*
intermittent fasting, *72*, 73–75, 137
inulin, *72*, 127, 146, 175

K
K cells, 118
Keys, Ancel, 97

L
LA (linoleic acid), 16, 66, 95–96. *See also* seed oils
L cells
   game plan for, 126–29, *128*
   GLP-1 drugs' effect on, 122–24, *123*
   gut conditions for, *8*, 19–21, *22*, 79, *84*, 113–20, *114–15*, *117*, *121*
   new paradigm for weight loss, 186

resistance training and, 127
Victory Checkpoint, 130
leaky gut
  Akker for, 75–76, 136
  overview, 14–15, *15*, 17–19, *19*, 85–86, 91–93
  reality check, 30
  seed oils and, 102–4
"lean mass" loss, 47–49, *48*
lifting weights, 49, 55, *55*, 56, 127
linoleic acid (LA), 16, 66, 95–96. *See also* seed oils
lipopolysaccharide (LPS), 14, 30, 66, 152–53, *153–54*
liver health, 66–67, 106, *107*

M

maculopathy (retinal damage), 47
malondialdehyde (MDA), 100
mental health signals, 50–51, *51*, 180
metabolites, 138–39, *138*, 148, 157, *158*, 159
Metchnikoff, Élie, 59–60, 186–87
Mounjaro. *See* weight-loss (GLP-1) drugs
mucin, 64–65, *64*, 75
mucus lining of intestines
  Akker's effect on, 4–6, *5*, 10, 60, 64–67, *64*, 75–76, *76*, *121*, 124–25, *125*, *153*
  fasting and, 73–74
  fiber and, *13*, 14, 155
  function of, 65, 86
  Gut Gems and, 86–87, *88*
  oxygen gradient for, 62, *63*, 102–3, *103*, *168*
  seed oils and, 19, *19*
muscle loss, 47–49, *48*

N

nonarteritic anterior ischemic optic neuropathy (NAION), 47

O

obesity, 17–18, *18*, 66–68, *69*, 97–98, *98*, 105–6, *107*, 124–26, *125*, *134*, 136

obligate anaerobes, 10–12, *11*. *See also* Akkermansia muciniphila; oxygen gradient

obstruction of intestines, 42, *43*

omega-3 fats, 109–10

omega-6 fats, 16, 109–10. *See also* seed oils

optic nerve inflammation (papillitis), 47

oxygen gradient, 10–12, *11*, 60–62, *61*, *63*, 88–91, *89*, 102–4, *103*, *105*, 119, 159–60, *160*, *168*

oxygen-intolerant gut microbes, 10–12, *11*. *See also* Akkermansia muciniphila; oxygen gradient

Ozempic. *See* weight-loss (GLP-1) drugs

Ozempic face, 3, 33, 42

P

pancreatitis, *43*, 44

papillitis (optic nerve inflammation), 47

partial stomach paralysis, 42

pasteurized Akker, 9–10, *9*, 21, 23–24, 70–71, 75, 124–27, *125*, 132–37, *134–35*, 171, 173

peptide YY (PYY)
  Akker and, 133, *135*
  fiber and, 151
  function of, 83, *84*, 118
  game plan for, 127
  L cells and, *114–15*, 116–18, *117*
  new paradigm for weight loss, 186
  overview, *8*, 20–21, *22*

physiological hypoxia, 89, *89*

P9 (protein), 20–21, *22*, 119–21, *121*

polyphenols, 30, 72–73, *72*, 157–59, *158*, 162–63, 174–75, *175*

postbiotics, 131–49. *See also* Akkermansia muciniphila
  delivery of, 25–27, *25*, *28*, 71, 132–36, *134–35*, 139–40, *140*

double-shield breakthrough, 141–45, *142–44*
integration routine, 145–48, *147*
mechanism of action, 136–40, *138*
overview, 22–24, *23*, 131–32
plan for introducing, 148–49
restoration protocol for, 171
prebiotics, 24, 68, 127, 146–47, *147*. *See also* fiber
pre-procedure checklist, with weight loss drugs, 49–50, *50*
probiotics
    Akker research, 70–72, 126 (*See also Akkermansia muciniphila*)
    "dead" probiotics, 131–49 (*See also* postbiotics)
    defined, 131
    delivery of, 25–27, *25*, *28*, 70–71
    function of, 24, 60
    integration routine, 146–47, *147*
    overview, *23*, 60
    restoration protocol for, 32, 167–68, 172–74, *173*
propionate, 5, 6–7, *7–8*, 82, *83–84*, 84–85, *88*, *117*, *164*
protein intake, 49, 55, *55*, 127, 161
Proteobacteria, 104, *105*
protocol. *See* restoration protocol
PYY. *See* peptide YY

R
regulatory T cells (Tregs), *83*, 84, 85
resistance training, 49, 55, *55*, 56, 127
resistant starch, 29–30, *29*, 155–57, 162, *163*, *164*
restoration protocol, 167–84
    expected outcomes, 178–80, 183
    GLP-1 drug comparison, 180–82
    overview, 31–33, *31*, 167–68, *168–69*, *182*, 183
    phase 1: barrier repair, *31*, 32, 169–72, *170*
    phase 2: reseeding, *31*, 32–33, 172–78, *173*, *175*, *178*
    Victory Checkpoint, 184
retinal damage (maculopathy), 47

retinopathy, 47
Roseburia, 76
Rybelsus. *See* weight-loss (GLP-1) drugs

S

safflower oil. *See* seed oils
SCFAs (short-chain fatty acid), 6–7, *7–8*. *See also* Gut Gems
secretory immunoglobulin A (sigA), 87
seed oils, 95–112
    chemistry, 98–101, *99*, *101*
    diet tweaks to support gut health, 108–12, *111*
    gut health effects, 101–4, *103*, *105*
    historical context, 96–98, *98*
    leaky gut linked to, 66, 86
    obesity and metabolic disease linked to, 105–8, *107*
    overview, 16–19, *17–19*, 95–96
    restoration protocol removal of, 169–72, *170*
Seed-Oil Sleuth, 108–9, 112
semaglutide. *See* weight-loss (GLP-1) drugs
short-chain fatty acid (SCFAs), 6–7, *7–8*. *See also* Gut Gems
sigA (secretory immunoglobulin A), 87
sleep, 17, *31*, 32, 171
soluble fiber, 28, *29*, 155–57, 164, *164*. *See also* fiber
soybean oil. *See* seed oils
spores (synthetic), 141–45, *142–44*
surgery and procedure precautions, with weight loss drugs, 49–50, *50*
"synbio" coatings, 27, *28*
synthetic "spores," 141–45, *142–44*

T

thyroid risk, *43*, 44
tight junctions. *See also* leaky gut
    Akker and, 65, *121*

colonocytes and, 5–6, 83, *84*, 85–86, *88*
fiber and, 153–54, *153*, *158*, 159, *160*
Gut Gems and, *7*, 13–14, *13*
lifestyle inputs and, *128*
seed oils and, 102–3, *103*
time-restricted eating (TRE), 73–75, 137
toll-like receptor 2 (TLR2), *64*, 65–66, 136–37, *153*, 155
toll-like receptor 4 (TLR4), 152–53, *153–54*
Tregs (regulatory T cells), *83*, 84, 85
Trulicity. *See* weight-loss (GLP-1) drugs
two-step protocol. *See* restoration protocol

U
ultra-processed foods, 100–101, *101*, 106, 111–12, *111*

V
vegetable oils. *See* seed oils
Victory Checkpoints, 34, 57–58, 78, 112, 130, 165–66, 184
vision risks, 45–47, *46*

W
waist-to-height ratio, 176, *178*
water intake, 171
Wegovy. *See* weight-loss (GLP-1) drugs
weight lifting, 49, 55, *55*, 56, 127
weight-loss (GLP-1) drugs, 35–58
   Akker comparison, 21–22
   alternatives, 54–56, *55*
   costs, coverage, and counterfeit problems, 52–53, *52*
   gut-derived GLP-1 comparison, 122–24, *123*
   hype versus evidence, 36–38, *37*, 57
   informed consent over hype, 57
   mechanism of action, 1–2, *2*, 38–39, *38*

muscle and bone loss, 47–49, *49*
overview, 35–36, *35*
real-world adherence and whiplash effect, 39–41, *40*, 53–54, *54*
restoration protocol comparison, 180–82
side effects (gallstones and bile duct issues), 44–45, *45*
side effects (general), 3–4, *3*, 41–42, *41*
side effects (mental health effects), 50–51, *51*
side effects (serious gut risks), 42–44, *43*, 46
side effects (vision risks), 45–47, *46*
surgery precautions, 49–50, *50*
Victory Checkpoint for, 57–58
Weight-Loss Conquests, 34, 57–58, 112, 130, 165–66, 184
weight-loss research and breakthroughs
Akker, 4–12, *5*, *7–9*, *11*, 59–78. *See also* Akkermansia muciniphila
fiber, 12–15, 28–31, 150–66. *See also* fiber
GLP-1 drug effects, 1–4, 35–58. *See also* weight-loss drugs
GLP-1 hormone and Akker's secret weapon, 19–22, *22*, 79–94, 113–30. *See also* GLP-1 (glucon-like peptide-1) hormone; L cells
modern fats research, 16–19, *17–19*, 95–112. *See also* seed oils
new paradigm for, 185–87
oxygen-intolerant gut microbes, *11*
postbiotics and postbiotic delivery, 22–27, *23*, *25*, *28*, 131–49. *See also* postbiotics; probiotics
science references, 189–237
two-phase plan for weight loss, 31–33, *31*, 167–84. *See also* restoration protocol
Victory Checkpoint for, 34, 57–58, 78, 112, 130, 165–66, 184